Enlightening Cinderella

Other works by Suzanne E. Harrill
(all published by Innerworks Publishing)

Books for Adults

Affirm Your Self Day by Day: Seed Thoughts for Loving Your Self

Affirm Your Self Daily Journal

Empowering You to Love Yourself

You Could Feel Good: A Self-Esteem Guide, Growing and Changing into Your True Self

Creating a Better You Teaching Manual: A Guide for Creating Greater Awareness, Sound Self-Esteem and Good Relationships

Cassette Tapes for Adults

Empower Your Self: Affirmations and Meditation

Building Self-Esteem

Books for Teens

Empowering Teens to Build Self-Esteem

Exploring * Connecting * Emerging: Adolescent Self-Esteem Curriculum

Children's Items

I Am a Star, My Building Self-Esteem Book

I Am a Star Self-Esteem Cards

Enlightening Cinderella

Beyond the Prince Charming Fantasy

By Suzanne E. Harrill

FINDHORN
Press

© Suzanne E. Harrill 2001

First published by Findhorn Press in 2001

ISBN 1-899171-58-4

British Library Cataloguing-in-Publication Data.
A catalogue record for this book is available from the British Library.

Library of Congress Catalog Card Number: 00-109405

Edited by Tony Mitton
Layout by Pam Bochel

Front cover design by Dale Vermeer

Printed and bound in Canada

Published by
Findhorn Press

The Park, Findhorn
Forres IV36 3TY
Scotland
Tel 01309 690582
Fax 01309 690036

P.O. Box 13939
Tallahassee
Florida 32317-3939, USA
Tel 850 893 2920
Fax 850 893 3442

e-mail info@findhornpress.com
findhornpress.com

This book is dedicated to my husband,

Rodney A. Harrill

I appreciate that you "stayed on the dance floor" with me over the years so I could transform my "inner Cinderella." I have grown so much since our dance-of-life began in 1965 at my high school senior prom. I am honored to learn with you how to dance a long-term, actualizing relationship.

And

our three wonderful daughters,

Lindy M. Johnson
Janna M. Shuemake
Sara C. Harrill

Acknowledgements

Many people assisted in bringing this book to fruition over several years.

To the people who have helped me with my creative process:

Thank you Karin Bogliolo, Publisher, Findhorn Press for believing in this book.

Thank you to my long-time friend, Diane Langley, for being there, helping me from day one and editing earlier versions.

A special thank you to Dianne Schilling for the professional editing that added spice to *Enlightening Cinderella*.

Thank you to Tony Mitton and Pam Bochel for the final polishing. Dale Vermeer, the cover is beautiful.

Table Of Contents

Introduction

We can discover many things about ourselves by examining our favorite fairy tale. My favorite is *Cinderella*.

For many years I found comfort in the magical belief, harbored by my inner child, that when circumstances became too difficult I would be swept off my feet by a handsome prince and rescued from all my problems. I nourished the fantasy that I would find the one person in all the world created just for me and that we would live together happily for the rest of our lives. Perfectly matched, we would enjoy instant rapport, an equitable, trusting, caring relationship, an absence of conflict, and absolutely no disappointments. Sound familiar?

Well, needless to say, it didn't work out that way. As an adult, living with my prince, I soon realized that life wasn't about luxuriating on a bed of pillows, daydreaming away endless carefree days devoid of challenges and conflicts. I eventually figured out that the only person responsible for creating my life was me, and that relinquishing all power to my mate put me on a path strewn with disappointment and frustration. Yet these issues — life authorship and personal power — have continued to challenge me. Not surprisingly, they are major issues for many of my clients as well.

Fairy Tale Symbolism

For many, the story of Cinderella nourishes the fantasy of finding a perfect partner — a Prince Charming. Symbolically, this fantasy represents the desire to integrate the inner self with God or the divine Self. One way to understand the inner self in this context is to see it comprised of both female and male parts. The less integrated these two parts, the less we understand ourselves and the more we project our need for fulfillment onto others, such as a fantasy prince or a "knight in shining armor."

Another interpretation of the Cinderella story asserts that the fairy tale is really about the heroine's (and by extension our own) quest for an "inner mother." According to this interpretation, Cinderella's father, prior to embarking on an extended business trip, asked each of his three daughters what gift she wished him to bring back. The two stepsisters asked for material things, while Cinderella asked for a branch from a hazelnut tree. Cinderella received the branch and planted it on the grave of her mother. Over the years, Cinderella's tears watered the branch and it grew into a hazelnut tree. This symbolizes the healing process Cinderella went through in grieving the unmothered child within and growing into her new life. At a very deep level, it represents learning to mother one's self. Many of us are involved in just this type of healing.

Catalysts for Healing

The underlying theme of *Enlightening Cinderella* is that we must heal ourselves and move beyond misconceptions about life and relationships that result from early childhood conditioning.

Throughout the book I remind the reader that relationships teach us about ourselves, and that events and conditions in the relationship are reflections of what is consciously and unconsciously inside of us. We live from our present level of awareness and we can only attract a partner similar to us in consciousness, with similar lessons to learn.

Through relationships we have the opportunity to heal the past, achieve personal mastery, express our unique life purpose, and grow into enlightenment. This process can take us beyond mere contentment and happiness to a place of joy and bliss.

Asking for Help

An important feature of the Cinderella story is often overlooked: Cinderella was able to connect to a spiritual being who loved and assisted her and, when necessary, performed magic. *Enlightening Cinderella* strongly illustrates the importance of the spiritual relationship that Cinderella had with her angelic helper, and emphasizes that this source of help is available to everyone. We are not alone. Spiritual helpers — angels, inner guides and teachers on more expanded planes of existence — are ready to assist when we get too far afield and cry for help.

In the fairy tale, Cinderella uses Fairy Godmother's powers to find an adoring husband willing to offer her security and prosperity. In *Enlightening Cinderella* other needs surface for Cinderella. Through Fairy Godmother's tutelage, she learns about the real opportunity offered by a love relationship, which is to know and love her true self. Once she recognizes that she is not a victim of life, Cinderella learns to consciously create what she wants to experience. She awakens to the deeper mysteries of life, and begins to understand why she was born and how to fulfill her unique purpose in life.

The Mirror Game

Partners in a relationship have reciprocal patterns that "plug into" each other. When two people meet, a process of engagement occurs to determine whether the two have anything in common that's worth exploring. Each person is like a sphere of energy with radiating rays. The spheres rotate, searching for mutual "docking points." When one is found, a bridge is opened between the pair and an attraction or chemistry is felt by both. This happens in intimate as well as non-intimate relationships. When two people have nothing in common, they pass each other and act as if the other does not exist in their world. There is no attraction. If a person is in your world, rest assured that the two of you share at least one growth issue, perhaps several.

We come to know ourselves by studying our reflection in the mirrors provided by others. Characteristics that we recognize and respond to in others reflect existing or potential parts of ourselves, though often we are unconscious of those parts. Qualities and behaviors we like and dislike in others give us feedback about our own psychological makeup. To grow and evolve, we select those aspects of our personalities that we want to keep (e.g. open-mindedness, curiosity, love) and weed out those we want to eliminate (e.g. prejudice, fear, being judgmental). Seeing traits in others allows us to make these choices.

What we do not accept in ourselves we project onto others. Projection is a defense mechanism where we protect ourselves from ourself when it is too painful to own certain traits, emotions, behaviors, or beliefs. Close relationships are the perfect ground on which to heal projections. Once the door of awareness opens and we stop denying what is inside of us, we can begin to accept and transform our shadow or unconscious side. We are then ready to live a more mature life and experience more mature loving relationships.

Projection is an important psychological construct that we need to understand if we are to gain access to hidden parts of ourselves. Characteristics and habits that we judge, avoid and criticize are easier to see in someone else than in ourselves. Seeing them in ourselves is too difficult. To begin healing we understand that what we see in another must reside within us too. We can thank our partners for reflecting back the unknown parts of ourselves that we refuse to face directly.

Projections do not have to be negative. We also disown such qualities as powerfulness, the ability to create money, nurturing, and certain emotions. Sometimes we react to opposing characteristics in others, yet deny that we play any part in the behavior pattern. For example, a neat, tidy, organized person ends up with a partner who is sloppy and disorganized. In dealing with issues of neatness and tidiness, both partners act out extremes. To begin working consciously with this situation, seek a middle-ground. For example, the neatnick begins to mitigate her own extreme behavior. Eventually, in response, her partner will move toward the center as well.

When we live with someone, we are faced with the need to heal and balance our past, including hurtful events, parenting deficiencies, and our attitudes and feelings toward caregivers. Our partner mirrors all kinds of unfinished business — from childhood, from former relationships, from belief patterns and from unprocessed feelings.

As issues with our partner surface, we have the opportunity to become more aware of deep seated influences, and to live our life in a more mature way. Many times our actions in the present are based on past experiences. If we are stuck in the past, relying on the perceptions of our wounded inner child, the people currently in our lives are apt to trigger negative responses. As we grow and heal, we learn to correct the misperceptions of the inner child, to live consciously, to integrate past and current experiences, and to reach a place of enlightened living. This latter state is characterized by the ability to problem solve, make wise choices, develop supportive relationships, communicate clearly and effectively, live with integrity and authenticity, and continually unfold in the process of actualizing our potential.

Loving Ourselves

Self-esteem is another important factor in spiritual growth and inner healing, one that is too often neglected or overlooked. If we do not love and nurture ourselves, we become needy, hoping someone else will fill us up. Life doesn't work this way, however. The degree we love ourselves determines our capacity to recognize love in others. We can only give and receive love based upon how we love and nurture ourselves.

To create good relationships we must start with knowing, accepting, and loving ourselves. The more we learn to love and forgive ourselves, the more that love becomes part of our relationships.

Loving ourselves includes looking at our negative side as well as our likable side. I had a client who spent two years in therapy leaving a bad marriage. Once she was out of the marriage she realized she could no longer blame her ex-husband for her negative issues. She was forced to own the controlling, angry parts of herself.

Because she was willing to look deeper, this client was able to heal some of the core issues that caused her to be unconsciously attracted to the type of man she rejected on a conscious level. She discovered how much she resembled her father, a man who held all the "bad guy" projections for her family of origin, and whom none in the family liked. Over time this client made peace with the angry and controlling parts of herself, forgave her father, and ceased to be attracted to men with these same qualities. She no longer unconsciously desired a partner on whom to project her own unacceptable traits. This client is now learning to love and nurture herself and hopes in the future to attract a loving and caring man.

Communication is Key

Basic communication rules and strategies also improve partner compatibility, and are among the lessons that Cinderella and Charming must learn in the story. They include:

- Open-mindedness. We need to keep in mind that there are always other points of view besides our own. Our partner's point of view makes perfect sense to him.

- Empathy. Putting ourself in our partner's shoes helps us to understand why he makes the choices he does.

- Listening. Most of us need help in this area. When we are triggered by something our partner says, listening stops and the mind closes while we wait to express our reactive thoughts and feelings. By spending time alone, we can often figure out the nature of the trigger issue so that when it comes up again we can listen.

- Risk taking. Some of us need to learn the art of loving confrontation and the skill of asserting our truth to our partner.

Putting the Pieces Together

We contribute to our relationships whatever degree of wholeness we have achieved. A whole relationship cannot be produced through a union of fractured partners. When we build the wholeness within, we build the potential of the relationship.

We need to work on our own insecurities (all people have them) and not make our partner responsible for filling those voids. At times our partner is able to provide exactly what we need, which can make a particular insecurity seem nonexistent. However, when our partner cannot meet the need, we must face the void and heal it.

Many therapeutic techniques are useful in that they can help us heal — for example, inner child work, visualizations, affirmations and journal writing. More important than any of these techniques, however, is the willingness to move to the spiritual level and experience the love and nurturing of a higher Source. Meditation is a good place to begin.

Measuring Progress

Unfinished business from childhood always shows up in adult relationships. Without realizing it, we take on our parents' patterns of thinking and behaving as well as social/cultural norms. It is important to see ourselves as a part of a family and a cultural system, and to realize that the improvements we make are built on the foundation of our conditioning within that system. My clients often become impatient with the long process required to create a good relationship. They set high goals for functioning in their relationship and feel disappointed when they don't measure up. I often urge clients to look back to where they started and measure their progress, rather than gauge the distance from their present reality to the ultimate goal. I help them to be loving and accepting both of themselves and the process. Goals are good because they give us direction; however, they must not be allowed to supplant present experience.

As a therapist, I see the following pattern repeated often. One partner, usually the female, feels pain and separation as the relationship "falls from grace." She is the catalyst for creating a genuine and authentic union. Whether or not she initiates some type of counseling, she begins to seek out and discover the path of healing and intimacy. Under ideal circumstances, she impacts her partner so that he, too, does the transformational work necessary for an enlightened relationship.

Let us learn about ourselves by looking at Cinderella ten years after her happily-ever-after marriage. As she experiences disillusionment and endures the pain of unhappiness and unfulfillment, Cinderella reaches a point of crisis which launches her inner journey. As our story begins, we find Cinderella in a garden behind the castle.

Chapter One

Ten Years Into Happily Ever After

Cinderella shivered and pulled the shawl securely around her shoulders. The April sky was blue, but the chill in the herb garden was numbing despite the shelter of heavy stone walls. Weeding and trimming would normally have kept Cinderella warm, but today she was too preoccupied to notice the new shoots of fresh dill, much less their pungent aroma.

Cinderella was twenty-nine years old. She and Prince Charming had just celebrated their tenth wedding anniversary, albeit not so happily.

Their storybook romance had unfolded quite smoothly during the first few years of marriage. In the beginning Cinderella's attention had been focused on moving to the castle. Soon she'd been occupied with adjusting to her duties, responsibilities and a higher standard of living, and, very quickly, to having and raising a family.

But obligations — even royal ones — don't distract forever. And, for some reason, Cinderella had chosen this day to squarely face reality and anxiously question her motives for marrying the prince.

"Is *this* living happily ever after?" she wondered. "Everyone else seems to think it is. I hear it over and over. My stepsisters and stepmother remind me practically every time we cross paths."

"No one would understand," Cinderella said aloud, pacing back and forth. "What possible excuse do I have for being unhappy? I live a lavish lifestyle in a luxurious castle. I'm up to my vaulted ceilings in gorgeous gowns, and have at least three-hundred pairs of glass slippers. More importantly, I have two wonderful children, and love being a mother. But in spite of all this, I feel terribly lonely, especially right after I've been around Charming. He always seems so happy and enthusiastic, running his kingdom and preparing for the day when he will be king.

Cinderella cried out in exasperation. "I don't have that kind of enthusiasm for *my* life! On the contrary, I feel as barren as a field after harvest, as empty as a pond in a drought. Charming doesn't excite me anymore, and I don't seem to turn him on either. He's obviously not the soulmate I thought I had found ten years ago, and I'm certainly not living happily ever after," she cried. "What's wrong? Why am I so miserable? What am I doing to deserve this? I need help!"

Cinderella stopped abruptly and glanced around to see if any of the castle staff had heard her frustrated outburst. Thankfully, she was alone.

She walked a little farther into the lush garden, past beds of primroses, cottage tulips, daylilies and glove pinks. She felt safer expressing her concerns where only the trees, flowers and animals could hear.

"Something feels different today," Cinderella mused, pivoting slowly, still unconvinced of her solitude.

Expecting to see Gosford the gardener or one of her children, Cinderella was startled to encounter her plump, elfish Fairy Godmother standing framed by a trellis of climbing roses and observing her quietly.

"My dear Cindy," said Fairy Godmother, extending her ample arms lovingly.

Squealing with astonishment and delight, Cinderella plunged through the flower beds and into the embrace of her celestial guardian, where she clung for several moments, jumping up and down and enveloping both in a pink cloud of falling rose petals.

"Where on earth have *you* been all these years?" cried Cinderella, finally stepping back.

"Well, actually, my dear, I haven't been 'on earth' at all. I've occasionally visited your dreams at night, and I've tried to work with you from a less worldly dimension. You haven't needed me to appear in person — or in *fairy* — until now."

Fairy Godmother backed up a little and appraised Cinderella carefully. "I wouldn't have come at all if you hadn't consciously asked — or should I say *yelled* — for help. The folks up at the castle may not have heard that outburst, but I certainly did."

Cinderella rolled her eyes and sighed heavily.

"It looks to me like you've reached a point of crisis in your life. Up until now, you've managed pretty well on your own. You've learned to be a good mother, that's for sure. How old are the children?"

"Marc will be eight in two months, and Mandy just turned five," answered Cinderella. "But they are not the source of my problems."

"Oh, I know that perfectly well," replied Fairy Godmother. "And neither is being a princess. In my opinion, you are handling the royal responsibilities of running the castle like a pro. And up until now, you've had a fairytale relationship with Charming, if you'll excuse the pun. Lately, though, you've been questioning very deeply. And you haven't been listening to my guidance, so — here I am," smiled Fairy Godmother warmly.

"How long can you stay?" asked Cinderella, as she picked her way out of the flower bed and back to the gravel path, leading Fairy Godmother by the hand. "Can you answer my questions before you go? Will I have to wait another ten years to see you again?"

"Wait a minute, wait a minute," Fairy Godmother laughed, scraping mud from her boots. "I'll get exhausted at this pace. Yes, we can talk now for as long as you wish. I'll try to give you insights into some of your dilemmas and answer many of your questions. And I'll continue to visit you here in this garden on a regular basis, until you have the situation in hand."

"Where do we begin?" demanded a relieved Cinderella. "I have *so* many questions. I need *so* much help. I am *soooo* unhappy."

"Why don't we begin with a discussion of soulmates," answered Fairy Godmother.

Cinderella smiled, "You really have been listening to me."

"Yes, well, you made napping fairly impossible," teased Fairy Godmother. Then with a deep breath that brought the fairy to her full four feet, she said, "We need to answer your question about whether Charming is your soulmate. Unhappiness has caused you much doubt, and you've been feeling disconnected from the marriage. We also need to talk about romantic love and its purpose in a relationship."

Cinderella's lips parted, but no sound emerged. She was astounded at her guardian's perceptiveness.

"First of all," continued Fairy Godmother, "I think you should understand that *soulmate* is a term you humans have invented to explain your desire to reawaken feelings of wholeness and completeness within yourselves. Since you identify primarily with the physical world," she declared with a sweeping gesture meant to take in the entire estate, "you tend to forget about the spiritual part of your nature. When you can't find fulfillment in yourself, you look for it in someone else — a husband, lover, or even a child. Which, by the way, diminishes your personal power."

"Really," was all Cinderella could manage.

"Feeling fulfilled by your mate's presence is wonderful and exhilarating, but when you expect this from your partner *all the time*, you set yourself up for disappointment. No one, not even the prince, can make you feel whole and gratified on a permanent basis. It's an illusion to think that he can be responsible for your emotional well-being. To truly be happy, you must find wholeness and emotional security within yourself."

Seeing Cinderella's look of bewilderment, she added, "And besides, most humans are in the same pickle as you are. Lacking complete self-awareness, they are not whole enough to give you what you want. Therefore it's folly to turn this responsibility over to the prince. He cannot possibly meet all of your emotional needs. Why he isn't even meeting his own!"

"I don't know if I follow you," said Cinderella. "And besides, Charming and I are very happy sometimes. I just wish we felt that way more often."

"Okay," reasoned Fairy Godmother. "Let's look at your situation as it is right now. Your unhappiness grows daily while the prince seems to be doing fine. He's busy and doesn't need you very much anymore. Is that your perception?"

Cinderella nodded slowly and lowered herself onto one of the stone benches lining the garden path. Her eyes misted slightly in response to Fairy Godmother's frank assessment.

"And is it also true that you feel your life is no longer good and satisfying because Charming doesn't give you the attention he once did?" The princess answered with another cautious nod as Fairy Godmother plunged ahead. "Frankly, I think you'd like to return to the grand ball. It was frantic and frightening in some ways, but it was certainly glamorous. Charming had you on a pedestal then and the relationship, if you can call it that, was pulsing with energy from all the infatuation and romance. Now that you are no longer the center of Charming's every waking moment, you assume that he must not be your soulmate. Am I right?"

"Yes, *yes* — to all you have said so far," responded Cinderella, deeply distressed. "I know it sounds selfish, but I'm terribly unhappy and I don't know what to do about it. And I don't understand what you are trying to tell me about wholeness. Don't I look whole to you?"

"I can't argue with you there," smiled Fairy Godmother. "What I'm trying to say is that you focus too much on the prince as the source of your happiness. But the prince is outside of you, and your happiness lies *inside* of you. I know this is a completely new idea. It will take time for you to reeducate yourself and grasp what I have to teach you. You can't slip into it like a dress or a pair of glass slippers. You must understand these ideas and make them your own."

"But that could take forever! I don't want this to consume a lot of time. Just give me something to make this tight feeling in my stomach go away! Can't you just wave your magic wand and say *abracadabra* or something?" implored Cinderella.

"No, my dear Cindy. The laws of this universe make it plain that you are in charge of your individual consciousness. You possess free will so that you can choose the rate of your own growth. No one can do that for you, not even me. However, I will gladly spend time helping you to understand yourself and correct your misperceptions about relationships. That lump in your stomach will ease over time," Fairy Godmother promised with authority.

"First, you need to understand how your family of origin — the family you grew up with — has influenced you. Second, you need to grieve the loss of your mother. Third, you must work through the emotional trauma of having been abused and exploited by your stepmother and stepsisters, and eventually forgive them. I'll help with all of those things," explained Fairy Godmother, plopping down next to Cinderella on the bench. She took Cinderella's hand and clasped it firmly in her own. "And that's just the beginning, my dear. That's just the beginning."

Cinderella squeezed her guardian's hand warmly in return, her eyes resting on the sundial that stood in the center of the garden. Her attention was suddenly seized by the deep shadow cast by its copper gnomon. "Heavens," she cried, jerking her hand away and jumping to her feet. "It's almost time for the children to have their dinner. I like to be there while they eat their evening meal, especially when Charming is away. We've been talking so intensely, I completely forgot my normal routine."

Fairy Godmother was already on her feet, adjusting her voluminous attire in preparation for a hasty departure. Flustered, Cinderella reached out and held her back. "I'm sorry, I mean it's *nearly* time for them to eat. I don't have to go inside *quite* yet. Please stay a little longer."

"No, my dear, we've made a good start and I really should be going," responded Fairy Godmother, "but I do have something to leave with you." Rummaging around in her bag, the old elf withdrew a beautiful rainbow-covered book. "Here, this is for you."

"It's beautiful," Cinderella exclaimed, opening the book, "but the pages are all blank. I don't understand."

"That, Cindy, is your first journal."

"Journal?" questioned Cinderella.

"Yes. I want you to write each day about your thoughts and feelings in reaction to the ideas we discuss. You will need a way to manage and make sense of everything that bubbles to the surface of your awareness as we talk. Currently your thoughts and feelings are churning around and around inside and you have no way of understanding or digesting them. Experiences, like food, need to be digested and metabolized. Fun and happy experiences assimilate easily, but painful ones, many just below the surface of your awareness, need to be brought forward and processed. Talking to me is one way to process significant emotional events. Writing in your journal each day is another."

"A simmering cauldron, that's me all right," laughed Cinderella. "I have a virtual stew of feelings inside. It keeps getting thicker and I do not know what to do about it. I'm willing to give anything a try."

Fairy Godmother was pleased. "Tonight when the children are in bed, simply take out your notebook and write whatever bubbles to the surface."

"Oh, the children. I've got to go."

"See you tomorrow, same time, Cindy?"

"Yes indeed," Cinderella called over her shoulder as she disappeared through her sitting room doors.

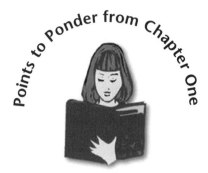

Points to Ponder from Chapter One

1. Spiritual insight, guidance, love, and nurturing are available to everyone.

   To begin the process and open the door to a new way of life, all you need do is ask. Help is always forthcoming, though the timetable may not match your perceived needs. For example, suppose you have a problem and begin to ask questions. Then you read an article in a magazine, pick up a self-help book in a bookstore, or catch a television program examining a similar problem. Perhaps a friend recommends a workshop or a therapist. You begin to find answers to your questions. You might experience some synchronistic event or circumstance that doesn't make sense at the time, but leads you on a new path. Perhaps you run into an old friend you haven't seen for years and learn that the path she is on fits your needs perfectly. You are being guided and directed because you opened yourself to greater awareness by asking for help.

2. When you are in emotional or spiritual crisis and ask for help, you always receive a spiritual response.

   You might have a vision or receive a silent message during meditation or at night in your dreams. Or guidance and love might come from beyond the physical world, such as through a guardian angel or spirit guide.

3. It is wrong to believe that if you are not infatuated and "in love," you are not with the right partner.

Many people cling to this misconception even when the partner was initially thought to be a perfect match.

4. Your happiness does not depend on being the center of your partner's life, as you were early in the relationship.

   Once the infatuation wears off, there's a tendency to think you are no longer in love and need to get away from your partner. But true happiness and fulfillment result from growing strong *within*, they never come from a partner.

5. It takes time and dedication to heal emotional wounds from the past and grow into wholeness.

   Until you learn to find emotional security and fulfillment within yourself, you may mistakenly believe that it can come from a partner. To truly live happily ever after, you must understand yourself and how to meet your own needs. A deeper search is required to answer such questions as, "Who am I?" and, "What are my needs?"

6. A relationship needs attention if it is to last beyond infatuation.

   There are no quick fixes for relationship problems. Healing takes time. Awareness builds mature love.

Journal Questions

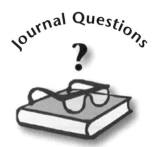

I suggest that you find your own "garden behind the castle" — a quiet place where you can be alone for short periods of time. Buy a notebook or "blank book" and use it to respond to the same questions that Cinderella is answering. Begin to develop a "blueprint" of your self. Over time, it may prove helpful to answer the same questions more than once. As you gain new information and insights, your answers will change and evolve. Occasionally, you will think of additional relevant questions. Write them down and answer them, too.

Don't be surprised if answers to some questions elude you at first. Some will not come easily. It is normal to experience frustration at the beginning of the healing process. It takes time to build the expertise to be the examiner of your own life. A close friend or counselor may be able to help you get started.

Answer the following questions to stimulate a deeper understanding of yourself. If you have a journal, write down your answers. If you do not have a journal, start one.

1. Under what circumstances do you get off track and find yourself wanting another person to fill you up emotionally, to make you feel whole and happy? What can you do differently to meet your own needs?

2. Describe your beliefs about trust and spiritual guidance. Where did you acquire these ideas? Do you need to update some of them? What has experience taught you?

3. Are you aware of your spiritual helpers? Are you open to receiving spiritual help? What do you need special help with today?

4. Do you have rituals or habits that allow for quiet time to study, journal write or meditate to connect with your spiritual self? How can you set the stage to receive spiritual guidance?

5. Write about thoughts, feelings, and reactions you had about the garden discussion topics.

Chapter Two

The Past Influences the Present

Cinderella and Fairy Godmother continued their visit in the garden the next afternoon. The sun was high and unfettered by clouds, prompting Cinderella to spread her shawl on a patch of lawn and stretch out to absorb the warm rays. The topic of discussion was the family of origin and its impact on current relationships. Fairy Godmother explained that Cinderella was probably still affected by the loss of her mother and the abuse of her stepmother.

"I can't believe I need to grieve the loss of my mother. She died years ago. I spent a lot of time writing about this last night in my journal. How could it possibly affect me now or have anything to do with my relationship with Charming?" asked Cinderella.

"Those are good questions," replied Fairy Godmother. "The simple answer is that people follow a natural process in coming to terms with the death of a loved one. The process doesn't vary much from person to person, and everyone needs to go through it, including you. If you *don't* go through it, the loss doesn't get resolved in your mind and heart. It resurfaces in various disguises and can cause a heap of trouble. For example, you may have developed hidden feelings of insecurity, or a fear of being abandoned. Those feelings cause you to react in certain ways when Charming isn't as charming as you'd like. Chances are your emotional responses and behaviors are way out of proportion to the situations that trigger them."

"If you mean I overreact," said Cinderella, "you're right. Sometimes I go off the deep end, making all kinds of accusations and needing lots of assurance, and then feel embarrassed afterwards."

"Well, take some comfort in knowing that you overreact for good reason," explained Fairy Godmother, adjusting wire-framed glasses on the bridge of her short nose. "Remember, you were very little when your mother died. You weren't much more than a baby, so no one thought it important to talk to you about your feelings. No one comforted you when you felt sad and lonely, or encouraged you to cry. No one held and rocked you when you were afraid or had a bad dream. When you felt angry at your mother for leaving you, there was no one willing to listen and understand. Your father did the best he could, but he was a very passive man. He didn't talk about feelings, and he wasn't particularly affectionate, although he did love you very much — more in fact than anyone else in his life. The reason he remarried so quickly was to create a better situation for you. Your father was quite naive and unaware when he married your stepmother."

Cinderella hugged her knees and squinted against the sun, her attention riveted on Fairy Godmother. She felt as if the old spirit was sifting through snapshots deep in her memory, shining a torch on events and conditions following her father's remarriage that even Cinderella had forgotten.

Fairy Godmother continued, "My guess is you didn't realize until now that you were abused by your stepmother. She never hit you, but she certainly misused her power as the adult in charge of taking care of you when your father was traveling. She punished you by withholding food and overworking you. That's physical abuse. She tried to humiliate you and hurt your feelings at every opportunity — clearly psychological abuse. And there was absolutely no nurturing. You are such a bright, loving soul, Cindy, I'm convinced your stepmother didn't do any permanent damage. However, you did suffer emotional wounding. Your intuitive connection with the animals and an ability to meditate protected your spirit and enabled you to ignore harsh, abusive conditions. In addition, the early years of love and nurturing helped you to tolerate the difficult passage caused by your mother's death."

Cinderella sighed, "You're right. It never occurred to me that I was abused by my stepmother. I'm beginning to see that her mistreatment, combined with my mother's death, might be affecting me in my relationship with Charming. But I still don't understand *how* it is affecting me."

Fairy Godmother's eyes twinkled. "I'm pleased that you are starting to consider these implications, but don't be in too big a rush," she cautioned. "It's probably going to take awhile to fully comprehend the impact of your childhood. Some people need a lifetime to sort things out."

"Oh, you mean I can't become an expert today?" asked Cinderella, feigning haughty impatience. Softly she added, "Actually, I want you to know how grateful I am that you are willing to spend so much time with me."

Yanking out a handkerchief, Fairy Godmother dabbed her eyes and polished her glasses fussily. "Yes, dear, I feel your appreciation," she said sternly while subjecting each lens to a painstaking inspection. Clearly, the old spirit loved her mortal charge very much.

Cinderella waited a respectful moment and then continued to describe her inner turmoil and conflicts with the prince. Fairy Godmother repositioned her glasses and listened intently.

"Right now I need some help resolving my problems with the prince. Let me give you some examples. First of all, Charming is very busy managing the kingdom and its assets. He makes important decisions every day, and loves it. I look at him riding off and feel useless, like I should be doing something as valuable with my time," said Cinderella. "Then there's my horse."

"Horse?" Fairy Godmother looked puzzled.

"Yes, horse. Charming gave me a champion gelding for my birthday last year. He loves the tournaments and wants me to compete with him — you know, be his partner. But I don't ride very well, much less race or jump, and I really don't like all that competitive stuff. The prince can't help but be disappointed in my performance. I'm always backing out at the last minute and letting him down. Once I even fell off the horse right in front of the reviewing stand. Winning is everything to him, but with me the only thing he wins is everyone's sympathy. I can't do anything worthwhile," complained the princess bitterly. "I guess I should try harder but..." Cinderella stopped abruptly and narrowed her eyes at Fairy Godmother. "Okay, I can see it in your face. You're thinking that this has nothing to do with my horse and riding fast, aren't you?"

"Dear me, I don't mean to be *that* transparent," chuckled Fairy Godmother. "But, yes, there is a deeper meaning to all of this, so let's stay with your examples. These situations are unpleasant because you are looking at them through the eyes of the person you think you *should* be. Always be aware of 'shoulds' and 'oughts'. Usually when you think you *should* be doing something, the value you place on the activity is not coming from within you. The value is coming from someone else. So rule number one is, pay attention to what *you* want and catch yourself when you think or say, 'I should...'"

Fairy Godmother continued, "You are a very giving person and derive a lot of pleasure from pleasing others, Cindy, so you may find it extremely difficult to tell the difference between what you really want and what others want for you. When you first stop doing a 'should' behavior, be prepared to feel mixed up for a while. Don't be surprised if you feel guilty about not pleasing Charming — or whomever it is. That will change. As you become convinced of the need to be your own authority, you will take risks and willingly pay the cost, whether positive or negative. Over time, your choices will become progressively wiser, more closely matching the desires of your true self."

After a moment, Fairy Godmother added, "By the way, you *are* capable of making decisions, managing money and winning tournaments. But you have to deem those things important and desire to do them in order to find them fulfilling. Merely thinking that they are more worthwhile than what you are doing now isn't enough. If you wish, I will help you figure out how to develop those skills. But right now I'm eager for you to learn more about what is inside of you. I want you to ask yourself some questions and take time to ponder the answers."

"What kind of questions?" asked Cinderella.

"Here's some paper. Write these down and spend some time this evening answering them," Fairy Godmother said, and proceeded to dictate the following five questions:

1. What are the most important ways for me to use my time today?

2. What do I feel is important in life?

3. What are my gifts and talents?

4. What are my needs, visions, wishes, hopes and dreams? What do I like to do?

5. What unique contributions do I make to my marriage and family and how do those contributions fulfill some of my needs?

Fairy Godmother added, "As long as you place more value on what the prince does to contribute to the family and the kingdom, and respect what he wants you to achieve more than your own desires, you can't possibly feel good about yourself."

"Charming has a vision of what you should be, but it may not match your inner self. You have a habit of pleasing him and depending on him for approval. As long as you allow Charming's gratification to be your primary source of satisfaction, instead of developing your own interests and talents, you will feel weak, dependent and unhappy. The fact that you let Charming decide what you should do with your time is an expression of your low self-esteem. And you will continue to have low self-esteem until the situation is reversed. When you understand your inner needs and strengths, you will correctly perceive your beauty and value in this family, and your potential in life as well.

Fairy Godmother paused to let her words sink in before elaborating further. "When you live your life pleasing others or depending upon others for fulfillment or for validation of your okayness, who *you* are gets lost. It gets buried under the expectations of others, or your misinterpretation of what they want from you. After a while you don't have a clue who you truly are."

Cinderella was awestruck. This oddly clad sprite knew her exceedingly well and expressed exactly what she had been feeling but could not say. "Go on," she urged excitedly.

"If you want to find fulfillment and live happily ever after, it is imperative that you learn to develop your own power, based on valuing who you are. This will take time. Letting your wish to please others, or your desire to be taken care of, dictate what you do with your time will not bring long-term fulfillment. Long-term fulfillment comes from being exactly who you were created to be. I want to help you discover your soul's blueprint. When you know yourself and consistently express that essence, you can be happy regardless of the whims of your partner or the ups and downs of the relationship."

"This is a lot to think about," responded Cinderella, pressing her fingertips to her temples as if to prevent the ideas from escaping. "But I want to know more — much more."

"Enough for now, my dear! You need time to assimilate these ideas," smiled Fairy Godmother.

"Just one more question, please?" interjected Cinderella quickly.

"And what might that be, Cindy?"

"Will the prince and I stay married?"

Fairy Godmother wisely replied, "Do you remember what I said yesterday about free will, Cindy? So you know I can't answer that." Then she smiled politely and said, "It's time I left you in solitude to think about what we have discussed. I suggest we meet tomorrow at the same time."

Cinderella scrambled to her feet just in time to embrace Fairy Godmother before she disappeared.

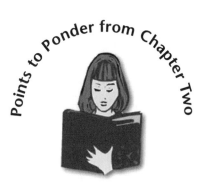

Points to Ponder from Chapter Two

1. Looking at your childhood and, in particular, your relationship with each of your parents, can help you to understand your current love relationship.

    If you are unhappy in your current relationship, your early years may afford clues as to why. It's important to determine how you were affected by the people who raised you.

2. Many of your beliefs about yourself and your relationships were learned from your family of origin.

    Your self-esteem developed in that context as well. So it's not surprising that your reactions to your current partner are based upon unresolved conflicts and patterns from childhood. For example, you may act out certain "scripts" with your current partner in order to get the love, approval and attention you failed to receive from your family. Things such as a divorce, death, the absence of a parent — even the abusive words and behaviors of adult caregivers — can affect you in adulthood.

3. Figure out what you want to do with your time.

    Stop making choices simply to please your partner or to gain love and approval. Likewise, stop doing things simply because you think you should. Only you can live your life.

4. Your self-esteem drops when you make your decisions based solely on pleasing others.

Stop shortchanging yourself. Instead of focusing on things you *should* be doing, envision things you *could* be doing and determine which of those feel right. Become your own authority and begin growing in the ability to make choices congruent with your inner self. Learn to be you.

5. Take charge of your life.

    No one but you can decide what is right for you. You may seek wisdom, guidance and assistance from others, but the responsibility to make choices is yours alone.

6. As you begin to discern and understand your true nature, take time to value your unique traits, interests and talents.

    This will empower you and build your self-worth.

7. Accept that dependency does not bring fulfillment.

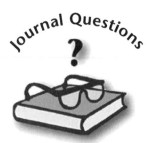

Journal Questions ?

1. Concentrate on your family of origin and list events, people, and patterns of thinking and behavior that may still be affecting you today.

2. List those things (activities, qualities, features, possessions, people) that you value in your day, your relationships and in your life as a whole.

3. What are your interests, gifts and talents? How might you develop and share them?

4. How do you contribute to the lives of others?

5. What do you want and need for your growth and development at this time in your life?

6. What are your private visions, wishes, hopes and dreams?

7. What do you like about yourself? What would you like to change?

8. What are some of your fears about yourself? How do they influence your life?

9. In what ways do you stop yourself from speaking and behaving in congruence with what you feel inside? When are you most likely to hide behind a mask?

10. In what areas of your life are you not being yourself and living your value system?

11. In what areas of your life are you afraid to take action and do what is right for you?

12. What is your most negative belief about yourself? Rewrite it to express what you know to be true. Continue this exercise to update your limiting beliefs.

Chapter Three

Beyond Romantic Love

For the rest of the evening, when she wasn't busy with the children, Cinderella did little else but write in her journal and think about her conversations of the past two days with Fairy Godmother. The prince was out of town for two weeks, negotiating water rights with five neighboring kingdoms. There was no pressure to share the garden experience with him because there was no opportunity, and for this Cinderella was grateful.

Fairy Godmother returned to the garden the next afternoon and found Cinderella in the private alcove off her sitting room, shielded from view by a thick curtain of honeysuckle and jasmine.

"Oh, Fairy Godmother, I'm glad you found me. I've been waiting for you!" exclaimed Cinderella, looking up.

"I know you have. I've watched you writing furiously in that journal. You've become as much a fixture in the garden as this bench you're sitting on," replied the wise old woman, plopping down beside Cinderella. They hugged and then relaxed for a few moments in silence.

"The more I write in my journal, the more questions come to mind," Cinderella said finally. "I wrote down some questions to ask you but they're not in any order and they don't make much sense at the moment, so I don't know where to start."

"Don't worry, Cindy. It's not necessary to share what you've written," responded Fairy Godmother. "The primary purpose of the journal is to develop awareness. Your questions will surface as needed during our time together."

Producing a small notebook from the layers of her gown, Fairy Godmother adjusted her glasses and quickly rifled through a dozen or so hand-written pages as if trying to find her place. "Let me see... if it's okay with you, I'd like to finish my explanation about soulmates," she announced at last, returning the notebook to its hidden depository.

Cinderella came to attention like an eager child on the first day of school. "Yes, of course, please do," she said.

"The term *soulmate* implies that one spiritual being or entity somehow produces two separate people who then become reunited when they meet and fall in love. This notion assumes that these spiritual twins satisfy all of each other's needs, accept each other totally, and never attempt to modify each other's behavior. Since the relationship is perfect, neither person has to confront the other or communicate deeper thoughts and feelings. After all, they can read each other's mind," asserted Fairy Godmother. "How boring!"

"But that's how it was for Prince Charming and me in the beginning of our relationship. And I loved it!" objected Cinderella.

Fairy Godmother raised her hand ever so slightly to quell the interruption. "I know, and we'll talk a little about romantic love in a minute. But, let me continue, please." Seeing Cinderella settle back, she resumed, "This type of relationship only works in a strictly spiritual dimension, which contains none of the day-to-day challenges and responsibilities of earthly life. In *this* life you have a personality with needs and wants and with appetites to satisfy, as well as a physical body to maintain. Daily problems and responsibilities create conflicts. Conflicts are not negative by the way, but normal when two people live together in the physical world. In a *true* soulmate relationship, the relating occurs strictly on the soul level, extending from your soul to the soul of your partner. The intention is to live from a higher plane of awareness while acknowledging that the physical world bestows its own special blend of challenges and lessons, such as the need to develop effective communication patterns and decision-making skills. Values, belief systems and experiences from each person's past are blended to create a totally unique relationship and family. Relating from the soul level is something you and the prince have yet to experience. It remains to be seen whether you are ready for that experience."

Cinderella could restrain herself no longer. "Wait a minute, please. How is a person supposed to know where spiritual relating leaves off and earthly relating begins? Should I sense a clear shift? Because I don't," she complained.

Fairy Godmother realized that perhaps she was delving too deep, too fast, and silently vowed to slow her pace to correspond with Cinderella's current level of awareness. As a teacher she was easily excited and sometimes gave more information than a mortal could reasonably be expected to digest. Her eyes swept over the garden's thick pink and purple carpet of April blossoms. On the other hand, she rationalized, it never hurt to plant an early seed or two. Like flowers, ideas tended to germinate in the right climate.

So Fairy Godmother listened while Cinderella endeavored to fathom the ideas she'd been presented with so far. Only when the rhythm of her recitation slowed and faltered did Fairy Godmother say gently, "You are digesting all of these new concepts very well."

"Thank you," said Cinderella. "But, you know, you're right about one thing. Grappling with all the everyday stuff has led me to believe that Charming and I aren't really soulmates. Now I'm starting to see some places where my thinking is flawed. I've been wanting fulfillment and haven't known how to find it within myself. I still don't. I've been disappointed that Charming no longer fills me up emotionally and makes me feel secure, when what I really want — as you've pointed out — is to be whole within myself. And I desperately want to relate to Charming from a soul level," finished Cinderella, her eyes clouding with tears.

"Cindy, tell me what you are feeling," urged Fairy Godmother.

"Well, to be honest, I feel very sad because I don't think Charming is in love with me anymore. I doubt that he would be interested in all this soul-relating business either."

"That doesn't matter, my dear," stated Fairy Godmother reassuringly.

Cinderella found her guardian's lack of concern upsetting. "Oh, yes, it does!" she objected. "I don't want to stay married to a man who isn't in love with me!" Now she was crying in earnest.

Fairy Godmother offered Cinderella a handkerchief. When the tears subsided, she tried to explain. "I see how upset you are, Cindy. Please don't jump to conclusions — I have a great deal more information to share with you. However for now, let's just focus on *you*. After all, *you* are the one sitting here eager to learn about yourself and your relationship."

Fairy Godmother leaned closer and said sagely, "I'll let you in on a little secret. It's so obvious that by now it shouldn't be a secret at all, but most people hide their heads from this one. *You can't really change another person, you can only change yourself.* When you do — change yourself, that is — the people in your life will either change in response to you, or they will eventually leave. Think of it this way: You are learning new 'dance steps' as you become more aware of yourself — of your expectations, needs, wants, behaviors, and reactions. And when you change the steps, Prince Charming will have no choice but to 'dance' with you differently."

Fairy Godmother continued, "Most of the men I've worked with feel much better being around a partner who knows herself, communicates without hidden agendas and game playing, and isn't expecting anything from them. And the same is true for women. In time, Charming may very well become curious about your transformation and decide to make changes in himself. But self-awareness is something only he can choose. And he is not sitting here talking to me right now."

Cinderella sighed heavily and said, "Well I'm here, and I definitely want to get to know myself, so I guess that means I'm going to learn some new dance steps. And I hope you're right about Charming dancing differently, too. But there are a couple of things I don't understand."

"What are they?" asked Fairy Godmother with raised eyebrows.

"Please explain what you mean by 'hidden agendas' and 'game playing,' because I'm not sure I understand," said Cinderella.

Fairy Godmother nodded approvingly. She liked the fact that Cinderella was paying attention to the subtleties of their conversation and thinking critically enough to ask questions. "A person with a hidden agenda seems to be trying to accomplish one thing, but is actually aiming for something else. That's why the 'agenda' is said to be 'hidden'. Sometimes the person with the hidden agenda doesn't even realize what she is doing. Her motives are subconscious. An example is a person who feels insecure and unloved, goes to her partner with a big hug and says 'I love you,' wanting the partner to hug back and say, 'I love you, too.' She appears to be giving love, but she's much more interested in *getting* love — and probably doesn't even realize it."

"Oh my, I do that all the time," admitted Cinderella.

"Game playing is similar. A game player is unwilling to be direct or straight with her partner because she believes her partner is incapable of responding to directness — that he will cut off discussion or get angry and refuse her requests. So she uses guilt, anger or charm to manipulate her partner, rather than tell the truth about what she wants and needs. For example, someone who is afraid to voice her opinions about how the money is spent may pretend that she doesn't care or is too scattered to pay attention to little details like overspending."

"Thank you — that helps," said Cinderella, getting up from the bench. She walked a few feet and stood beneath a large Hazelnut tree, gazing up at its lush branches. "My father planted a tree like this for me when I was about six years old," she recalled. "I used to sneak away from my stepmother and huddle under the tree when my father was away. I felt safe crying there. I guess I was looking for protection and security."

Cinderella ran her hand along the trunk of the tree. After a moment she turned to face Fairy Godmother. "Oh, how I wish the prince and I could return to our newlywed days. Everything was so perfect. He listened to every word I said and asked me lots of questions. He wanted to know all about me — my thoughts, feelings, everything. I was the center of Charming's world and I miss that."

Fairy Godmother could see they needed a little break, so she joined Cinderella in reminiscing about happier times, starting with her first appearance prior to the fateful grand ball. Eventually this led — as the old spirit knew it would — back to the subject of romantic love, whereupon she sat down again and smoothly resumed her teaching role.

Romantic love, she explained, was how most relationships began. The strong physical and emotional attraction between two people produced an altered state of consciousness that was not easily sustained past the infatuation stage.

"Chemicals in the brain called *endorphins* cause feelings of pleasure. At the beginning of a relationship, the couple's brains are saturated with endorphins creating this special state of infatuation. People get a similar feeling of well-being if they exercise vigorously or, would you believe, when they eat chocolate," grinned Fairy Godmother. The word "chocolate" seemed to make her ample body shudder ever so slightly.

"In this intense emotional state, your images, expectations and ideals of the perfect mate are projected onto your partner. These projections may have very little to do with who the partner really is. But it's hard to tell because both of you are on your best behavior. Joy, laughter, and attentiveness bring out the best, don't you think?"

"I certainly do," sighed Cinderella.

"In the beginning of the relationship, you and Charming were reeling with romance and passion, so responding to each other was easy. In addition, many of your emotional dependency needs were being met. You felt safe and secure both physically and emotionally. The deep loss of love you had experienced as a child, especially when your mother died, made the impact even greater."

Cinderella nodded her head repeatedly, and said, "I see without realizing it, I was seeking from Prince Charming the emotional security that I had not experienced since my mother's death."

"That's right, Cindy!"

"Everyone thought that all the riches of royal life were making me happy," said Cinderella, shaking her head sadly.

Fairy Godmother took the thought a little further. "These outer riches, however, never met your *inner* needs," she said softly.

"No. And I realized that more and more as the newness of the marriage wore off. I had what everyone else wanted and still wasn't happy. I felt that I had no right to be *unhappy*. What a confusing time it was."

"It was difficult to watch you suppress your pain and put on a happy face for others. You almost had *yourself* convinced at times," said Fairy Godmother.

"Why didn't you come visit me then?" asked Cinderella with the barest trace of resentment.

"Oh, I was tempted to rescue you. As a matter of fact, I was beside you the entire time, waiting for you to ask for help. It's very rare to intervene in someone's life the way I did in the beginning. I only jumped in because it was your destiny to be at the grand ball and that crazy stepmother of yours had you locked up. You have a very special purpose in life that required you to meet Prince Charming — but we'll talk about that later."

"I can see by the look on your face that I'll have to wait quite awhile for that revelation," smiled Cinderella. She walked slowly back to the stone bench and reclaimed her seat beside Fairy Godmother. "So.... getting back to our original discussion, why was I so unhappy?"

"Because Charming's willingness to provide the emotional security you were looking for was limited," Fairy Godmother answered. "He spent a lot of time with you during the first couple of years, didn't he?"

"Yes, he was very passionate and affectionate. We made love all the time. He frequently came back to the castle in the middle of the day to surprise me with flowers or a gift, and of course we always ended up in bed. He was available whenever I wanted to *talk*, too," added Cinderella as if to ease her embarrassment.

"You saw the best side of Charming during the early years of your marriage," Fairy Godmother explained. "He could only maintain that side during the romantic-love stage of the relationship, however, while he was infatuated. He relished your dependency on him because he was obsessed with you. But eventually, as his infatuation faded, he grew tired of the dependency. He felt trapped and smothered by it. Your dependency may have reminded him unconsciously of his relationship with his mother. She doted on him as a child, wanted to know everything he was thinking and every detail of his days. If he did not want to spend time with her, she pouted. He learned to distance himself emotionally and separate himself from his mother's smothering. When he was around his mother, he "checked out" so to speak. Physically he was there, but mentally he was somewhere else. He could daydream while looking her in the face, and even repeat her words if questioned. He survived by being emotionally cool, distant, and aloof."

Fairy Godmother stood and stepped back to study Cinderella, as though uncertain how to phrase her next statement. "Charming slowly pulled away from you when you started to remind him of his mother. He returned to managing the kingdom and resumed his training to be king. You interpreted this withdrawal to mean he was less in love with you. What looked like an expanding horizon to him represented emotional distance to you."

Cinderella nodded her head and added, "Sometimes when I tried to get close, he told me to quit acting like his mother. He accused me of using attention and affection to try to control him. Of course I took it personally. I was convinced that something must be wrong with me, that if I were a better wife he'd go back to being the prince I fell in love with. I can see now that he, too, has plenty of unmet needs from his childhood. His past affects our relationship, too."

"Yes, yes, you're right," replied Fairy Godmother, pacing back and forth on the dirt path. "You were able to maintain the facade of marital bliss by using childhood survival skills. To stay clear of your stepmother's rage, you always did what was asked of you and rarely listened to your inner needs and feelings. Of course, no amount of work was ever enough, nor was it possible to do any task to your stepmother's satisfaction. You learned to check out emotionally and live in a fantasy world of your own while waiting for your father's return."

Cinderella took up the story. "When Charming was no longer infatuated with me and returned to running his kingdom, I needed to check out in the same way I did as a child. I spent hours alone in the garden. Occasionally, the joy returned to our marriage. The births of Marc and Mandy were wonderful times. I spent long hours with my babies, practically oblivious to anything else that was happening. Actually, Charming was very affectionate when the children were infants. I truly felt loved at those times," said Cinderella, smiling again.

She continued, "As the children grew more independent, I occasionally became sad and depressed. I didn't understand why until now. I'm embarrassed to realize how many subtle, needy messages I've been sending to Charming. With all my demands for closeness, it's no wonder he feels overwhelmed. The only thing he knows how to do is distance himself emotionally."

Fairy Godmother had been listening in amazement to Cinderella's insightful observations. "I'm so happy that some of these issues are starting to make sense to you. When you can see the big picture, you don't have to take everything so personally or feel like a victim. You can create a new life for yourself and learn the secrets of truly living happily ever after," she said.

"I'm excited about all of this, too. But it almost sounds as though it is expected that love will die when two people in a relationship find out who they really are," observed Cinderella.

"No, I'm saying that love grows and changes. The love that emerges is very different," replied Fairy Godmother.

"What do you mean?"

"Well, do you remember when you and Charming began to quarrel frequently? You both started experiencing a lot of tension in the relationship," said Fairy Godmother.

"Yes, how could I forget? That's when I began questioning what I was doing here and doubting whether or not we were right for each other, or really in love," commented Cinderella. "In fact, there were times, I'm ashamed to say, when I didn't even *like* Charming anymore."

Fairy Godmother smiled and replied, "Here's a very important piece of information, Cindy. It was his *behavior* you didn't like, not his *inner essence* or *true self*. He could no longer be what you wanted him to be because he had another side you didn't know. He had needs that were not being met. To understand Charming, you have to look beyond his behaviors to see what's motivating him. At the time, for instance, he may have returned to the jousting scene because he needed more physical activity. Or maybe he needed more time to run the castle or prepare for his competitive tournaments. He had stopped doing those things when you were first married. To ease his guilt over not spending time with you, he strongly encouraged your riding lessons and entered you in tournaments. You stopped some of *your* activities, too, like meditating and talking with the animals."

Cinderella showed no signs of tiring as Fairy Godmother continued her discourse on relationships. The old expert explained that as infatuation and romantic love subside, a very important stage emerges. Healthy relationships go through a period of continuing power struggles. During this stage, each partner tries to mold the other into the "ideal" mate. As part of this process, many couples bicker and fight. Some launch a "cold war" and start avoiding the more sensitive areas of conflict. Since neither Cinderella nor Charming were ready to risk confrontation, their lives had become more and more separate and devoid of intimacy and sharing. They avoided conflict, at some level agreeing not to argue and fight openly. Yet the tension and pain remained, even without confrontation.

"You tried to suppress your negative feelings," concluded Fairy Godmother. "Until now, that is."

"Thank goodness you came back, Fairy Godmother," said Cinderella. "I've been feeling so cut off from life, much as I did when my father went away on business trips and I was left with my stepmother and stepsisters feeling like a prisoner in my own home. I'm relieved to understand that it's normal to fall out of romantic love and to experience conflict. If I hadn't been so afraid to confront Charming, I might have put some of this on the table sooner. I can see now that Charming and I have used guilt and blame to try to control each other in our effort to recapture feelings we had in the earliest stage of our relationship. We both longed for that period of infatuation when being together was new and exciting. I've missed the romance."

Cinderella's eyes softened as she recalled: "I used to fantasize as a girl about being the wife of a handsome prince. I imagined total, mutual dedication with nothing but blissful moments for the rest of our lives. In my fantasy, we were together all the time, enjoying the same activities, laughing, sharing our innermost thoughts and feelings and making love every day of the week. We discussed our roles as parents and agreed on how to raise the children. We sat together each evening watching our children laugh and play together. We studied and read books together and talked about life and philosophy. We enjoyed growing together." Cinderella stared at the perfectly manicured hedgerows. "Well, I'm sure you get the picture," she said. "I wanted my life with Charming to resemble that fantasy, which was pretty unrealistic."

"Yes, it was," responded Fairy Godmother, "but almost every newlywed has the same unrealistic expectation. And it does no good to tell couples what's ahead, because they refuse to believe that their ecstasy won't last. So besides being exciting and intoxicating, romantic love serves the very important purpose of bringing couples together.

Fairy Godmother began to search the folds of her gown distractedly. "I'm pleased that you are developing a deeper understanding of relationships. It's time for me to leave for today, but first let me give you a new set of questions to write about in your journal."

With a triumphant flourish, Fairy Godmother produced the following questions, hugged Cinderella and was gone.

1. List characteristics you like and dislike about your partner, including roles, attitudes, beliefs, habits and values. Which are characteristics that you also possess?

2. List characteristics you think your partner likes and dislikes about you. Confirm your list by sharing it with your partner. Note similarities and differences between the two lists.

3. List characteristics, interests, values and beliefs that you and Prince Charming have in common. List those that are in conflict. Clarify with the prince.

4. Write a poem expressing your current thoughts and feelings.

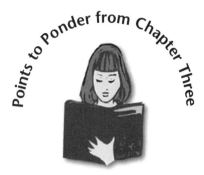

Points to Ponder from Chapter Three

1. A relationship cannot remain in the infatuation stage
    indefinitely.

    The ebbing of romantic love should not be construed as a signal
    that you are in the wrong relationship or have a serious
    problem. Romantic love is not mature love.

2. Dissatisfaction occurs in a relationship when the infatuation wears
    off and disillusionment sets in.

    Two people are now ready to blend personalities and learn to live
    together in true partnership. Areas of friction indicate problems
    that need to be solved.

3. Confrontation builds understanding.

    The second stage of a relationship is tantamount to an extended
    power struggle. This is normal. Learning to confront at this stage
    is healthy and helps the relationship mature. It allows each
    person to learn how s/he impacts the other. The challenge at
    this stage is to find out what can be changed in the relationship
    and what must be accepted.

4. In a mature love relationship, partners learn to relate on a soul
    level with considerable awareness.

    They understand that unfinished business from either person's
    past can show up in the relationship, and that early life
    experiences must be healed. Mature partners believe that they

are together for specific reasons and take time to discover and understand the purpose of their union. They are also aware that it is normal to have difficulties when two personalities are learning to accept each other and form a healthy relationship.

5. Self-awareness is the key to improving a relationship.

    Over time, increasing self-awareness will enable you to identify the hidden agendas and the games being played between you and your partner, and to develop new patterns of relating. Game playing and hidden agendas kill love.

6. You can only change yourself in a relationship.

    Changing your partner must never be the goal. Put your focus where you have control, which is with yourself.

7. As you change your own patterns of thinking, behaving and communicating, you automatically change the pattern of the "dance" with your partner. When you introduce new "dance steps," your partner will have to behave differently, too.

8. Each person in the relationship projects unmet expectations and needs onto the other, which causes misunderstandings and conflict.

    Aware partners eventually learn to recognize these projections and withdraw them in order to relate to the other person's true self. A projection is a psychological defense mechanism that enables a person to recognize characteristics in others that she is unwilling or unable to face in herself. A person must possess at least the germ of a characteristic in order to recognize the same characteristic in someone else.

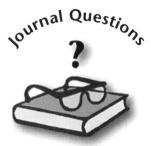

Answer the questions Fairy Godmother gave to Cinderella.

Chapter Four

The Building of Self-Awareness

Crouched in the herb garden, trowel in hand, Cinderella was imposing needed territorial limits on the oregano, which seemed intent upon overrunning its neighbor — and Cinderella's favorite herb — the basil. She looked up and laughed at the sight of Fairy Godmother struggling to untangle herself from a thorny rose bush. "You really must be more careful where you materialize," she admonished, peeling off her soiled garden gloves to offer assistance.

"I know, I know," huffed a vexed Fairy Godmother, examining one of several snags in her skirt. "I keep forgetting how thoroughly planted your gardener keeps the grounds — it's hard to find a safe place to land."

Cinderella led Fairy Godmother to an elaborate iron table installed only that morning in her private alcove. She had grown quite comfortable with the sessions in the garden and wished to provide equally comfortable physical amenities. As they settled into cushioned chairs, Cinderella remarked that they had met almost daily for two weeks.

"It is so consoling to have you back in my life. Writing in my journal is immensely rewarding! I've been writing poetry for a long time, but have never simply written about my problems — which, by the way, don't seem as overwhelming as they did last week or last year."

"I'm glad things are looking better. Recording your thoughts and feelings about an issue almost always has that effect," responded Fairy Godmother.

"I really have to concentrate when I answer your questions," continued Cinderella, "But by writing, I can get enough distance from the issues to think about them more clearly, which helps me to achieve greater balance. I'm developing some clarity and objectivity about my relationship with Charming, too."

"Good, good," said Fairy Godmother, nodding affirmingly.

"You know, when I first started answering your questions in my journal, I had some problems," recalled Cinderella. "For some reason, I wanted my writing to make sense to other people. I corrected my spelling and took a long time with the mechanics. Then, on a couple of your questions I had so many ideas that I wrote very quickly. I didn't have time to worry about my spelling and handwriting. Now I'm more at ease just letting my thoughts flow. Sometimes what I've written doesn't even make sense when I reread it a few days later — but that's okay because it made sense at the time, and I felt much better after expressing myself."

Fairy Godmother's enthusiastic nodding was by now rocking her chair perilously.

"Would you like to see some of my poetry?" Cinderella asked uncertainly.

"Yes, very much, Cindy, thank you for trusting me," Fairy Godmother encouraged.

"I have three I'd like to share with you," Cinderella stated, sliding a notebook in front of her companion. Fairy Godmother opened the notebook and began reading.

I REMEMBER

It is you I ask, as I cry silently,
To be there for me.
To be strong,
To touch me and
To hold me,
So I will feel secure.
When in reality,
I yearn
For that place inside of me.
Now I remember how
It is supposed to be.
You are not the one
To fill
Me up.
It must come
From the soul of
My Being.
I release the pain of
Feeling
Separate from you.
I heal from within
And trust instead
That the spirit
Within me will
Reveal true security,
LOVE from the
Source of me.
I now am nourished,
Filled from within.

THE PENDULUM

You leave as I approach.
I see my need for closeness
Pushes you away.
Gently I learn that what I need
You cannot give,
At least not at this time.
You ask for distance,
I ask for closeness.
The solution is for one
Of us to give what the other asks.
Since you need space, I will withdraw.
As I leave, you approach.
I turn around and we face
Each other.
For a moment, the pendulum
Does not swing.

I AM CLEAR

I let you go so I can be free.
For so long this strange paradox I did not see.
The bondage of holding on only trapped me.
I am clear now to let go and simply be.

Fairy Godmother put the notebook aside and applauded enthusiastically. Her radiant smile could easily have lighted the dark side of the moon. "You are touching your true self and your writing demonstrates much healing and wisdom. I recommend that you reread these poems during times of stress when everything you've learned seems to escape you. I'm very proud of you," she beamed.

"I can't wait for Charming to come home!" Cinderella exclaimed. "He'll be back in three days and I have so much to share. He's not going to believe it when he sees I'm back to my old happy and enthusiastic self."

As Cinderella talked excitedly about the pending reunion with her husband, Fairy Godmother kept most of her thoughts to herself. She wondered how she could warn Cinderella, who was so energized and had such good intentions, that there might be a bigger hill yet to climb. The prince didn't know, for example, that he was in the middle of a problem that affected the entire family system. If asked, he would probably say that his greatest difficulty was simply having an unhappy wife. He did not view *himself* as having a problem and he wasn't looking for answers. He hadn't even asked any questions.

Fairy Godmother doubted that Charming was aware of the degree to which living together creates interdependence. What one person does or feels affects the other members of the family. What's more, every family member is usually contributing in some way to problems like Cinderella's, often unconsciously. So the solution also has to involve the entire family.

Fairy Godmother decided to treat the subject cautiously for the time being and said, "Cindy, I share your eagerness to have the prince fully informed about our lessons. But I advise you to take it easy when you present your new ideas and insights. Don't share everything with him at once. After all, you have had a little time to digest these concepts."

"Oh, yes, I'm sure you're right. I'll be careful. Charming's going to be so excited that you're back in my life."

"Well now," was all Fairy Godmother could muster. It was clear that Cinderella was in no mood to have her excitement muted.

The two sat quietly for a few minutes, each pursuing her own thoughts. Finally Cinderella announced, "I'm ready to get on with today's lesson."

Without consulting her notebook, Fairy Godmother plunged into the day's subject. "Let's talk more about the growth of relationships," she said.

"That would be just great," replied Cinderella openly.

"After the first stage, infatuation, and the second stage, power struggles, comes a third stage in relationships, which is *unconditional acceptance*. At this stage, each person becomes highly aware of various traits in the other. Some you like and others you loathe, but you learn to accept the ones that can't be changed. Keep in mind that at times the second and third stages blend, so conflict and power struggles are not necessarily over at this point. In fact it is healthy at this stage to deliberately bring up areas of conflict in order to work them through to resolution or acceptance. As in the second stage, a couple needs practical everyday help, such as important communication tools that help to solve problems, resolve conflicts and process emotional reactions. The use of such tools enables a couple to correct the parts of the relationship that are amenable to change. With good communication, this can be a very fulfilling time in a relationship, with an abundant exchange of unconditional love and acceptance."

"It must be very gratifying to live from a place where you accept your partner unconditionally, without trying to change his basic nature," commented Cinderella.

"Yes, and a great deal of self-awareness is required to ensure that you each take responsibility for understanding your emotional reactions and needs and for getting those needs met," said Fairy Godmother. "By the way, the development of self-awareness is the main reason for all the journal questions."

"I can see that," agreed Cinderella.

Fairy Godmother continued. "You and your partner must each learn to express what you want and need. Then, *together* you go through the process of figuring out which needs can and cannot be met by the other person. This is a time when expectations are readjusted and both people become more realistic. Part of the process involves grieving the loss of expectations that cannot be met, and forgiving your partner for not conforming to your ideals. Making peace with yourself over the loss of your idealistic fantasies can take years — it really depends on how self-aware you are, and how tuned in to the relationship. At this stage, you let go of control and discover that it feels good to practice unconditional love and acceptance."

Fairy Godmother noticed that Cinderella's expression had grown increasingly troubled. She leaned forward to indicate her readiness to listen.

"That sounds good," the princess said sadly, "but I don't understand how this third stage is possible for us. We aren't even close anymore, and we certainly don't communicate well. I wouldn't know how to start."

"I see what you mean," responded Fairy Godmother, "and I don't mean to imply that moving from the second to the third stage is easy. But, my dear, you have already come a long way. Many people never understand enough to ask for help."

Fairy Godmother abandoned her chair and began walking around the table. Rounding out her fifth orbit she announced resolutely, "I think that as soon as Charming gets used to the idea that things are changing, we should invite him to join our garden discussions."

"Include Charming?" cried Cinderella jumping to her feet. "That's a wonderful idea. Oh, I wish he were home tonight. I hope he agrees to meet with us."

"Even if he doesn't, I can continue to teach you. The learning will eventually reach Charming — when *you* change the dance, remember? Whether he comes to our garden talks or not, there's still a lot of work that you must do. Mere understanding does not automatically heal emotional pain or correct unrealistic expectations. For some, a lifetime of lessons is needed to master unconditional acceptance."

Fairy Godmother reminded Cinderella firmly, "Even if Charming does join our discussions, remember that you and I are focusing on *your* healing and *your* goals. If Charming wants to work on himself and the relationship, that's fine. I will emphasize self-awareness and communication whether he comes to our garden sessions or not. Sometimes you will see progress, and other times you'll feel like nothing is working and the relationship has no hope of getting past the power struggles. So expect lots of ups and downs. Growing in awareness as a couple can be very slow. You mustn't expect rapid change."

Fairy Godmother took Cinderella's hands in hers. "I believe enough has been said for today, my dear."

"I think you're right," agreed Cinderella. "I want to get back to the children. What are my journal questions for today?"

"Ah yes, the questions! I came prepared with a new list for you," she said, and with a flourish waved a sheet of parchment in the air. When she vanished, it floated gently to the table.

1. List three things that frustrate or disturb you and that you wish you could discuss with your partner. Express your feelings. Share this list with your partner when the time feels right.

2. Do you have memories of experiences with Charming that still upset you? List the incidents for which you have difficulty forgiving your partner. What do you need in order to let go of these bad feelings?

3. Using your understanding of a mature love relationship, describe how you would like your relationship to be in five years time.

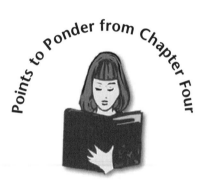

Points to Ponder from Chapter Four

1. Writing about your problems brings clarity, objectivity and a sense of relief.

    When you put your thoughts on paper, you do not have to keep mulling them over. Having a quiet mind reduces stress so that you can better manage your problems. Writing to express and understand your inner conflicts feels good and balances the emotions. It doesn't matter whether you write poetry, random thoughts and feelings, or letters that are never delivered, the effect is the same. Journal writing is not about reporting daily events but, rather, your *reaction* to each day's events or memories from your past.

2. If you are participating in therapy, attending self-discovery classes or reading self-help books, you need to slow your pace and temper your enthusiasm when interacting with a partner who is not involved in similar activities.

   A partner who is not seeking change will feel threatened and unsafe when significant change occurs around him.

3. Awareness of problems always precedes their resolution.

   Change occurs more slowly than ideas about change. Likewise, understanding does not automatically heal emotional pain or change patterns of behavior.

4. In its third stage, a healthy relationship moves beyond power struggles and control issues to unconditional love and acceptance.

   However, during the transition from stage two to stage three, partners must still confront and resolve issues in the relationship. This means taking risks to make positive change wherever possible and accepting those conditions that cannot be changed. Even in stage three, it is healthy to discuss anything that upsets you. Differences are approached positively, not as things to brush over, hide or suppress.

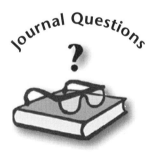

Journal Questions ?

Answer the questions Fairy Godmother gave to Cinderella.

Chapter Five

Life is a Process

Cinderella rushed out of the castle to find Fairy Godmother already in the garden. Clearly agitated, she gave her guardian a quick hug and began, "Do you mind if we walk? I really had a hard time sleeping last night after answering those journal questions you gave me yesterday. I was restless and lay awake for hours re-experiencing every negative feeling I've had for the past ten years. When I tried to think about mature love and how I want to be in the future, I just got angry. I don't see how this can work for Charming and me."

Unruffled, Fairy Godmother fell in with Cinderella's rapid stride. Clearly, the princess was feeling overwhelmed by her growing awareness, so the old elf simply listened for a time to her frustrated ranting. When there was a lengthy pause, Fairy Godmother said, "Believe it or not, Cindy, it's healthy to experience the stored anger that you have not allowed yourself to feel for the past ten years. I think perhaps you judge anger to be inconsistent with your warm, loving personality, but, believe me, it's okay to fume and fester sometimes. You don't have to be afraid of what you judge to be negative feelings and you don't have to let those feelings drag you down into depression. You can experience and release them by venting to me. It takes a lot of energy to deny what you feel. One goal of our meetings is to help you identify and acknowledge *all* emotions as you experience them."

Cinderella slowed her pace and spoke in a discouraged voice. "I don't *want* to deal with my anger — it's too difficult! Besides, doing all the things you suggest will take forever."

Fairy Godmother replied, "Not forever, my dear, but it will take time."

"How long?"

"That depends. It takes as long as it takes. Sometimes many years are required to deal with feelings, and other times the shift is made quickly. Cindy, I know you don't want to hear it right now, but I must emphasize that this entire transformation you are going through takes time." Fairy Godmother spoke gently but firmly.

"But I want it now, not in a lifetime," sighed Cinderella.

"Remember, this is a process," said Fairy Godmother, who had talked many times about the process of life being more important than the destination. "It is the journey of your life right now, today, that is important. It is always right now. Goals, when achieved, only satisfy for a short time. The nature of humans is to grow and strive and create, always moving on to the next goal and the next. It's naive to think that you'll be happy when a certain time in the future arrives. You are just getting started on the journey of living in higher consciousness. Try not to judge the process."

"But how can Charming and I overcome years of emotional separation?" asked Cinderella. "Change requires so much work."

"Yes, it is a lot of work, but time will go by whether you do the work or not. Imagine things staying pretty much the same and then look five years into the future. What does it feel like?" asked Fairy Godmother.

"Heavy," replied Cinderella.

"Now imagine devoting time and attention to these issues and picture the situation five years from now. How does *that* feel?"

"Light," smiled Cinderella. "You're right, I really must go forward and meet these challenges even if it's difficult and slow-going at times."

Fairy Godmother smiled breathlessly. "Can we stop walking for a few minutes?" she asked. "I want to explain how change works, and I'd like do it from a stationary position. Don't forget, you're a few centuries younger than I."

"Sorry," said Cinderella. "We can sit under this oak." She led her guardian a short distance from the path. They sat down on the soft grass facing each other.

Fairy Godmother began, "Let's look at your tendency to expect too much too fast while ignoring the process. Take a deep breath now and try to project yourself into the future. Pretend that for several months you and the prince have been talking and working actively to improve your relationship. Sometimes you do a very good job. You allow the prince to be himself, and you put into practice all the things we work on in our garden meetings. Then, out of the blue, an unhealed part of you surfaces. Maybe you feel insecure after running into your stepmother in the village. Temporarily, you forget that this insecurity is coming from within, and you repeat behaviors that you know will not produce the results you want. You demand more of the prince's time and try to make him feel guilty for traveling to tournaments and working long hours. This flips him right back into the old pattern of pulling away from you emotionally. Charming neglects to tell you how he feels. At the same time, he doesn't want to meet any of your needs for closeness. He checks out mentally, even when he's here physically, repeating his early pattern with his mother."

"It's pretty hopeless if we still do these things even when we have the information to act differently," said Cinderella, dubiously.

Fairy Godmother was quick to respond. "No, Cindy, you miss my point. I am saying that in the healing process you have to stand up and fall down many times before you learn to glide through the new steps. Each time you dance the wrong steps, one of you will eventually remember to do it the new way. Over time, as you create healthier and happier ways of relating and getting your needs met, you will spend less and less time repeating unfulfilling patterns. I can't stress enough that this takes time — like learning to play a musical instrument. No one ever taught you this, so I'm not surprised that you feel discouraged."

Fairy Godmother decided to take a new tack. "Cindy, what is one of the main purposes of a relationship, beyond meeting the needs of both partners and making sure the children are provided for?" she asked. "I alluded to that at our first meeting."

"What?"

"To help people to learn and grow in awareness. Life is a journey. Each person is in the process of becoming totally aware and conscious of their true inner self. Relationships provide a context in which to grow. People who choose not to live with a life partner tend to learn more slowly. Living with someone accelerates the pace. Your lessons are 'in your face,' so to speak."

She explained further. "You and Prince Charming were drawn to each other like magnets. You have reciprocal patterns to work out and balance during this lifetime. You have the opportunity to transform these patterns by 'dancing' with each other. 'The Dance of Life' is a good metaphor for the patterns occurring between you and Charming."

"I know some of my lessons," said Cinderella impatiently. "I need to forgive the past, to feel my feelings, to become strong within myself and not depend on Charming for my happiness. Tell me some of Charming's lessons."

"Okay, Cindy, but only because I want you to know that he has issues to confront, too. You are not the only one with problems. However, I don't want you to focus on Charming's lessons. After this discussion, I will keep reminding you to think *only* about your own," said Fairy Godmother.

She continued, "Charming has a pattern of wanting to rescue and provide material security, and then feeling he has been taken advantage of. He tends to take on too much responsibility. Currently he confronts both of these issues, yet is unaware of the fact. He interprets them as your needing too much and his doing everything for you. He does not see his part in the pattern."

"He most certainly does *not* do everything for me," protested Cinderella indignantly. "That's really unfair!"

Fairy Godmother responded reassuringly to Cinderella's defensiveness. "You and I know that he *chooses* to do these things for you. We also know that you handle many responsibilities quite competently without his assistance. But that's how *he* feels when he wants to change the pattern and doesn't know how. In an unhealthy way, he gets a little relief by making you feel guilty. Not too good a method is it, Cindy?"

Cinderella relaxed in response to her guardian's acquittal. "Thank you. I feel a little better. I was starting to feel guilty listening to your descriptions of the drama between Charming and me. I hate the thought that Charming believes I take advantage of him."

"I know, Cindy," comforted Fairy Godmother. "By the way, Charming probably would like to do many of the things that he criticizes you for doing. He would like to be taken care of. He might like to get out of some of his duties as a provider. He has much to learn about his own dependency needs and how he ignores them. Charming has developed a coping mechanism to handle uncomfortable feelings. When he starts feeling uneasy, he gets busy and keeps moving."

"So we both have issues with security and nurturing," summarized Cinderella.

"Yes. I think you are both looking for a deeper level of security, one that comes from feeling secure within. That kind of security can only result from connecting to your spiritual essence. Your patterns of excessive dependency and of looking for total security in Prince Charming fit nicely with his patterns of feeling trapped and moving away emotionally. In fact, they are reciprocal patterns — they plug into each other. Although it doesn't feel very good when these patterns surface, they provide you with a means of helping each other grow in consciousness. Each of you acts out perfectly the behaviors needed to 'trigger' the other into higher growth and awareness."

Cinderella stood and brushed grass cuttings from her dress. "I really want to grow secure from within myself," she said resolutely. "And strong, like this oak."

Fairy Godmother picked an acorn from the ground and held it out to Cinderella. "Here, my dear, " she said. "Why don't you keep this as a symbol of the oak tree's inner strength." With her extended hand she beckoned Cinderella to help her stand up. "The next time we meet, we will talk more about this inner power. I have some information to give you about how to build a strong foundation of self-esteem. Operating from high self-esteem makes it much easier to manage your insecurities and misguided thinking," she promised. "In time you will no longer expect the prince to take care of you. You will grow in your ability to mother yourself. This will upset the equilibrium of the relationship for a while, though. Then the see-saw will need to re-balance, this time with healthier patterns of relating. Eventually, I suspect that the prince will subconsciously sense your growing independence and find it safe to pull closer to you again emotionally."

"I appreciate your optimism," laughed Cinderella happily.

"I find it fascinating to watch the patterns and dance steps between partners," said Fairy Godmother as they strolled back to the garden path. "There are so many patterns to understand and heal. Eventually, both you and Charming will realize that you are whole and complete beings and in this relationship by choice. The relationship is the vehicle that transports you to this awareness and supports each of you on your life journey."

"Wow, this is quite a process," said Cinderella. They both laughed. Cinderella's use of the word *process* showed that her awareness had already taken a significant leap.

"I'm getting tired," sighed the princess. "I have enough to think about for now. But I could use a theme to write about in my journal. Please give me something that will help me focus on the ideas you've just described and use them."

"That's a very good idea. Write these down in your journal," said Fairy Godmother. She dictated three questions as they walked back to the castle.

1. Look at problems you are experiencing and patterns that repeat themselves, and use them to describe lessons that you are working on in life.

2. List possible reciprocal lessons that you and your partner are working on and explain how they fit together.

3. List lessons that you have already learned with your partner.

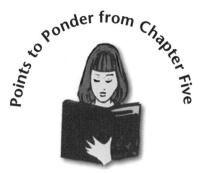

Points to Ponder from Chapter Five

1. Life is a process. We never get "there."

    Don't be in such a hurry to solve your problems that you miss the present moment. Just when you think you've arrived, you will discover new issues and want to set additional goals. So remember, this is it — this moment. The process of life is more important than the goal. Satisfaction comes from enjoying "right now" as you proceed toward your goals.

2. When you are in a fast growth cycle, expect wide mood and attitude swings.

    For a while you may be very much involved in the healing process, achieving a high level of understanding and change. Then, without warning, you may feel awash with frustration and find yourself resisting the entire process. It is time to pause and rest for a while.

3. One purpose of a relationship is to teach people about themselves, to help both partners grow in awareness.

    People are attracted to each other in part because of reciprocal patterns. These patterns create complementary life lessons that a couple can learn together. Relationships work better when partners understand that they have chosen the relationship because of unconscious patterns that need healing.

4. Unresolved conflicts from the past will show up in the relationship.

These provide opportunities to identify where growth is needed. Not all couples are able to weather changes generated by expanding awareness and freedom from old conditioning. Sometimes one partner grows and changes while the other remains unwilling or incapable.

5. The marital drama is like a dance.

    At first, most people feel victimized by traits and behaviors in their partner that they don't like. This victim role is willingly abandoned when they recognize and take responsibility for the lessons they have to learn. As one or both partners become conscious of the dance, they are able to risk new steps and the dance changes.

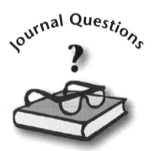

Journal Questions

I encourage you to open *your* journal and write any thoughts or feelings that came up while you were reading this chapter. Answer the questions given to Cinderella. In addition, describe issues pertaining to your relationship that you and your partner have decided to stop talking about. These are clues to the identity of unhealed patterns and opportunities for healing.

Chapter Six

An Introduction to Personal Power

Fairy Godmother arrived in the garden to witness Cinderella in animated conversation with one of the castle gardeners. The princess waved her guardian in the direction of the alcove table and indicated that she would join her in a couple of minutes.

The old sprite busied herself by sprinkling fairy dust on the marigolds, turning them red, then violet, then azure, and finally back to yellow. She was about to try silver when Cinderella slipped under the honeysuckle canopy and hurried to the table. Fairy Godmother quickly stashed the fairy dust and welcomed Cinderella with outstretched arms. The hug filled them both with heartfelt warmth and love.

"Gosford and I are planning a new greenhouse — nothing but orchids," she said, radiating a lightness Fairy Godmother had not seen before. "Learning about myself is surprisingly energizing — and there's so much more inside to know. I answered your questions last night and immediately thought of several others to ask myself."

Fairy Godmother was pleased. She had been watching Cinderella for many years, waiting for an opportune time to guide the young woman deeper into self-understanding and mastery. The princess was finally able to focus on herself rather than view her problems as stemming from her relationship with Prince Charming. It was an important step.

"Well, I'm ready for more teachings," announced Cinderella as they both sat down at the table.

"Are you indeed?" laughed Fairy Godmother. Cinderella conveyed an innocent, direct approach that she found endearing. "As a matter of fact, I have a very special lesson for you today. It may be the most important information we ever discuss."

"And what is that?" questioned Cinderella.

"I want you to understand about your personal power," replied Fairy Godmother.

Cinderella looked a little deflated. "I don't really like the word *power* and it scares me to think of being personally powerful."

"I know. And that is exactly why this is such important information. Just listen for a while and stay open to hearing what I have to say," said Fairy Godmother.

"That's fair. I'm all ears," smiled Cinderella, pulling her chair closer to the table.

"You, *and only you*, are in charge of your life," Fairy Godmother began. "Now that you are an adult, you are responsible for all the choices in your life, even the ones you make unconsciously or think that someone, like Charming, is making for you."

"You make choices based upon your belief system. In fact, you have a set of beliefs that guide your life. They function like rules. However, many of them are false beliefs that need to be updated in order for you to feel better emotionally. For example, you make many of your choices based upon the belief that you must honor Charming's wishes concerning your time and activities. You think that this lifestyle — these riches and comforts — are a direct result of his having chosen you as the perfect partner. You believe at a deep level that you would not have a husband or an abundant lifestyle without him — that you are powerless without him and unworthy without his love."

"That is probably true," nodded Cinderella. "And I suppose you are implying that I am powerful regardless of whether or not Charming is in my life. I have the right to make choices but have never given myself permission to make them."

"Yes. That's precisely what I'm suggesting. And as we work together, I think you will choose to rewrite many of your limiting beliefs. Which brings me to the subject of self-esteem." The forceful way Fairy Godmother said the words left no doubt that the crux of the day's lesson was at hand.

"Your self-esteem, which serves as the very foundation of your life, is a reflection of how well you love and accept your true self. When I say your 'true self' I am not referring to the conditioned self of childhood, or to your actions, or to who you think you *should* be. Your true self is your *spiritual essence* — who you are deep inside, on a spiritual level. Only *you* can be you. Your job is to remember the blueprint of your soul and to express it to the best of your abilities. As you grow in awareness, you will learn that you have the personal power to live an abundant, creative, loving, exciting life — with or without Prince Charming."

Cinderella nodded slowly. "That sounds like a monumental task, but it gives me a better understanding of what you mean by personal power. I was afraid that perhaps you wanted me to become daring and aggressive, which does not feel at all like me. To be exactly what I am created to be sounds perfect. Now I guess you'll tell me how."

"I'm glad you could hear the message and not get hung up on the words," said Fairy Godmother. "To begin with, I'd like to explain more about self-esteem. Then we can look at some beliefs that get in the way of having healthy self-esteem. Finally, I'd like you to become familiar with some signs of low, as well as high, self-esteem."

"Okay," Cinderella replied. "Let's get started."

"As I have said, self-esteem is how you feel about yourself. You consciously and unconsciously send thoughts and opinions *about* yourself *to* yourself. These thoughts can be accurate and helpful or they can be false and damaging. To build self-esteem, you need to use *self-talk* to consciously think and say positive, honest things to yourself in your mind. You may already hear negative self-talk and know what I am talking about. It's possible you've internalized the words of people from your past, many of which are damaging," explained Fairy Godmother.

"As a matter of fact, I believe I have," agreed Cinderella. "I distinctly hear my stepmother saying, 'You don't deserve to be a princess. It will never last. Prince Charming doesn't really love you. You aren't good enough to be royalty, you should be cleaning floors. The marriage will never last. He will get tired of you once he finds out what you are really like.' I used to be furious at her for saying such mean things, but deep down I thought maybe she was right. I have always doubted myself. I guess the memory of my mother's loving messages has grown too faint to override my stepmother's dismal estimation of me."

"Good example," replied Fairy Godmother. "Without your realizing it, those hurtful words of your stepmother have been alive in your mind, influencing everything you create in your life. Unfortunately, as long as a part of you believes what she said, you'll feel unworthy of receiving more from your relationship. You'll believe you don't deserve it."

Slowly, she added, "The good news is, you are at a place in your life where you can reprogram or *re-parent* your subconscious mind. You can correct the incorrect beliefs, assumptions, and messages you send to yourself."

"How do I do that?"

"Start paying attention to the manner in which you talk to yourself. Begin writing down statements and phrases that you hear mentally and that you suspect are neither true nor good for you. Then rewrite those statements. The revised statements are called *affirmations*. To heal your wounded consciousness, you must say the affirmations to yourself many times, and with all the feeling in your heart," explained Fairy Godmother.

"Please give me an example," requested Cinderella.

"Okay. Take the statement, 'I don't deserve all that Charming provides' or 'I am not good enough for Charming.' Change these to 'I deserve love no matter what' and 'I am a good and worthy person'. Many repetitions are necessary to change negative beliefs to positive ones. This approach is empowering and will enable you to make decisions based on a stronger, healthier belief system. You have to be a detective to uncover the false beliefs that guide your consciousness. Sometimes it's difficult to pinpoint them, and you may need my help occasionally. You have many beliefs that need strengthening, too."

"This is an assignment that requires vigilance," responded Cinderella thoughtfully, "and I believe I possess that quality. Tell me more."

"Now that is speaking from your place of power," cheered Fairy Godmother and they both laughed out loud.

"I'm getting it," smiled Cinderella.

"Now let me give you an important list which defines some characteristics that indicate low self-esteem. You will recognize some of them — you've seen them in yourself and others. Any extreme thought, feeling or action is a clue to the presence of low self-esteem." She then materialized a piece of paper with the following list:

Signs of Low Self-Esteem

- Self-blame and self-criticism, or constantly putting others down through guilt, blame, shame, faultfinding or gossip.

- Over- or under-achieving, eating, working, doing, etc.

- Remaining a victim, rationalizing that outside circumstances are the cause of your problems.

- Not taking responsibility for your own life; turning power over to another to make decisions for you, then feeling victimized if the results are not to your liking.

- Taking undue responsibility for the lives of others; dominating others and making decisions for them.

- Fear of change and reluctance to take risks; or frequently making changes thoughtlessly; taking dangerous, unwise risks.

- Constant negativity, or being so optimistic as to deny reality.

- Reacting to others with extreme emotion or with no emotion.

- Boastful, overbearing behavior around others, or inability to maintain integrity while interacting with others.

- Demanding to be "right," needing to have others' agreement or your own way most of the time, or constantly acquiescing in other people's will and opinions.

- Constantly comparing yourself to others; feeling inferior or superior.

- Black-white, either-or thinking, e.g. thinking a person's behavior makes them either good and valuable or bad and unworthy.

- Living from a place of fear, terror, or panic.

- Speaking with lots of shoulds, oughts, could haves, and yes buts.

- Interpreting the hurtful words or actions of others as proof of your unworthiness.

"Boy, I can sure see a lot of these in myself," Cinderella remarked pensively. "And my stepmother must really have low self-esteem. I think she has all of these characteristics and a few more besides."

"Yes, Cindy, that's right," said Fairy Godmother

"I suppose I should feel some compassion for her," added the princess.

Fairy Godmother nodded her head in agreement as she handed Cinderella another sheet of paper and patiently watched her read.

Signs of High Self-Esteem

- Having an internal locus of control, getting "okayness" from within.

- Taking care of self physically, emotionally, mentally and spiritually.

- Having ability to balance extremes in thoughts, feelings and behaviors; and when out-of-balance, taking the necessary action to correct.

- Learning from mistakes and being able to say, "I made a mistake, I'm sorry."

- Managing your life responsibly.

- Honoring individual differences among people.

- Listening to other points of view.

- Taking responsibility for your own perceptions and reactions; not projecting onto others.

- Being able to listen to your wise inner self, or intuition, and to act on this guidance.

- Having self-respect, self-confidence and self-acceptance.

- Having awareness of your own strengths and weaknesses.

- Choosing continuous self-improvement and taking positive risks.

- Balancing being and doing.

- Feeling warm and loving towards self.

- Being able to give and receive love.

When Cinderella finished reading, Fairy Godmother continued. "In summary, high self-esteem is a feeling of total acceptance and love for yourself *as you are*. It means respecting and valuing yourself as a worthwhile human being. It means seeing your good and not-so-good qualities honestly. And it means taking care of and nurturing yourself so you can grow and become all you are capable of being. High self-esteem is a quiet, comfortable place where you enjoy and accept who you truly are."

Fairy Godmother pushed her chair back from the table and folded her hands in her lap. The two sat quietly for a few moments.

"Before I leave," said Fairy Godmother, standing up, "I want to give you a tool to help you understand more about self-esteem. It's called the Self-Esteem Inventory. Each of the twenty-five questions is intended to catalyze your thinking. They also make excellent affirmations to update your belief system. You may want to write in your journal about the areas where you score low. Another good technique is to copy the statements on small pieces of paper and stick them around the castle as reminders to repeat them often. I want you to have several days to work with these ideas before we meet again."

"All right, I'll spend some time on these things over the next few days," promised Cinderella. "This was an unusual lesson. I imagine the information will be very helpful when we talk about my relationship with Charming again."

Fairy Godmother smiled, realizing that Cinderella still found it easier to concentrate on Charming and the relationship than on herself. She handed Cinderella the Self-Esteem Inventory, scheduled a meeting the following week, blew a kiss and was gone.

Cinderella sat down in the garden and began pondering her answers to the Self-Esteem Inventory.

The Harrill Self-Esteem Inventory

Rate yourself on a scale of 0 to 4 based upon your current feelings and behaviors:

0 = I never think, feel or behave this way.
1 = I do less than half the time
2 = I do 50% of the time
3 = I do more than half the time
4 = I always think, feel or behave this way.

Score   **Self-esteem Statements**

1. I like and accept myself right now, even as I grow and evolve.

2. I am worthy simply for who I am, not what I do. I do not have to earn my worthiness.

3. I get my needs met before meeting the wants of others. I balance my needs with those of my partner and family.

4. I easily release negative feelings when other people blame or criticize me.

5. I always tell myself the truth about what I am feeling.

6. I am incomparable and stop comparing myself with other people.

7. I feel of equal value to other people, regardless of my performance, looks, IQ, achievements or possessions (or lack of them).

8. I take responsibility for my feelings, thoughts, emotions, and actions. I do not give others credit or blame for how I feel, think, or what I do.

9. I learn and grow from my mistakes, rather than use them to confirm my unworthiness.

10. I nurture myself with kind, supportive self-talk.

11. I love, respect and honor myself.

12. I accept other people as they are, even when they do not meet my expectations, or their behaviors/beliefs are not to my liking.

13. I am not responsible for anyone else's actions, needs, thoughts, moods or feelings, only for my own (exception, my own young children).

14. I feel my own feelings and think my own thoughts, even when those around me think or feel differently.

15. I am kind to myself and do not use "shoulds" and "oughts" to put myself down with value judgments.

16. I allow others to have their own interpretation and experience of me and realize that I cannot control their perceptions and opinions of me.

17. I face my fears and insecurities and take appropriate steps to heal and grow.

18. I forgive myself and others for making mistakes and being unaware.

19. I accept responsibility for my perceptions of others and for my response to them.

20. I do not dominate others or allow others to dominate me.

21. I am my own authority. I make decisions with the intention of furthering my own and others' best interests.

22. I find meaning and have purpose in my life.

23. I balance giving and receiving in my life. I have good boundaries with others.

24. I am responsible for changing what I do not like in my life.

25. I choose to love and respect all human beings regardless of their beliefs and actions. I can love others without having an active relationship with them.

This is not a test. Neither is it a precise measure of self-esteem. Its purpose is to identify beliefs that affect self-esteem and may need modifying. Place no judgments on your score. Consider taking the indicator every six months to gauge your progress. Low numbers indicate beliefs and patterns that may block you from loving and feeling good about yourself. All of the statements make good affirmations. To change negative beliefs, repeat the statements to yourself regularly. Use the indicator to help you understand other people, too. Recognizing that someone whose behavior you find unacceptable has a self-esteem problem makes compassion and forgiveness more accessible.

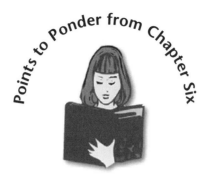

Points to Ponder from Chapter Six

1. Personal power comes from a strong foundation of self-esteem
    and requires that you take responsibility for your life.

    You are responsible for the choices you make, even the ones that
    are made unconsciously or are turned over to others.

2. You make choices consciously and unconsciously based on your
    belief system.

    Many beliefs that guide you are invalid or immature, yet they
    affect your choices and the day-to-day results you experience.
    Outdated beliefs require updating.

3. Self-empowerment is built on a foundation of healthy self-
    esteem.

    Extreme thoughts, feelings and behaviors are signs of low self-
    esteem. High self-esteem is the quiet, comfortable state of
    enjoying and accepting who you are. It is characterized by the
    congruence between inner and outer states.

    It is important to learn to love and accept yourself and take
    responsibility for your level of awareness. The Self-Esteem
    Inventory provides a means of looking at beliefs that affect your
    self-esteem. To improve how you feel about yourself, update
    negative beliefs.

4. Become aware of your self-talk. Replace negative with positive
    statements, and speak to yourself in a kind, loving and
    supportive voice.

Create positive affirmations to update your guiding beliefs and repeat them to yourself regularly to reprogram your subconscious mind. Affirmations gradually replace the negative conditioning from childhood that you have internalized in the form of negative self-talk. As your beliefs about yourself improve, so will your feelings about yourself improve.

5. Who you really are is neither the conditioned self from the past nor the person you think you should be. The unique person you really are is a manifestation of your spiritual essence or true self.

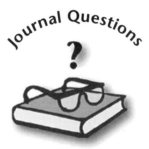

Journal Questions

After taking and scoring the Self-Esteem Inventory, write down your thoughts and feelings about areas in which you gave yourself a low score.

Chapter Seven

Mirrors and Polarities

It was evident that the past few weeks had been good for Cinderella. Her excitement was infectious, and before long the entire castle staff waited breathlessly for each visit from Fairy Godmother. It was obvious to everyone that the princess thrived in the company of this feisty old spirit who cared about and nurtured her.

Cinderella was beginning to understand the impact of many of her life experiences. Deep inside some of the pain still lurked, but somehow it didn't matter as much because Cinderella was grasping the lessons behind the pain. She was seeing the bigger picture of how life works and internalizing ideas and information that helped her heal and change. This made the pain bearable.

Cinderella's bountiful energy and reconnection to life was having a positive influence on just about everything and everyone. Everyone, that is, except her husband, Prince Charming.

Fairy Godmother tried to help her protégé understand why Charming was having difficulty accepting a happy, enthusiastic wife.

"Our lesson today is about relating emotionally to your husband, Cindy," began Fairy Godmother, as she settled back in her chair at the alcove table.

Cinderella was systematically plucking dead blooms from the alcove plants. "Good," she responded firmly, without looking up. "He really confuses me. Until recently, I was unhappy — even depressed — about practically everything. Now that I'm starting to laugh again and connect with everyone, the prince gives me stern looks and pulls away. I don't understand it. I thought he more than anyone would be elated to see me happy again."

Lightheartedly, the princess tossed a handful of camellia petals into the air, proclaiming, "I *am* happy! In fact, most of the time I feel so good inside I go around singing and dancing." She demonstrated with a catena of quick steps and a graceful pirouette. "The staff tell me I positively glow. Then I spend time with Charming and, for some reason that I do not understand, I come away feeling sad and disappointed." Cinderella sank into a chair, her mood suddenly changing. Her eyes brimmed with tears as she privately recalled events of the previous evening.

"You see? Look at me starting to cry. I feel jubilant one moment and miserable the next. A few nights ago I tried to explain to Charming some of the ideas I've been learning from you. I told him that I'm working on becoming more independent and not needing him as much. And you know what? He wasn't interested. Oh, he *said* he was, but he didn't really listen. He was polite, but kept looking at the hour glass and leaning towards the door. Since then, whenever the prince and I have been together and I've broached the subject of my experiences with you, the results have always been the same. You told me to go slowly, but this is ridiculous. I've only told him a little, and it's obviously too much for him."

"That's okay, dear. At least he knows something's up. It's better to do a poor job communicating than to keep him completely in the dark."

"Well I must be doing a poor job," sighed Cinderella. "He did say he would come to the garden. But I must warn you there was little enthusiasm in his voice and it will be another week or so before he can fit us into his schedule. That disappoints me, because I want you to explain all these ideas to him as soon as possible."

"I understand your need to move things along, but it's great news that he's willing to be here *at all*. And we can still continue *your* lessons," smiled Fairy Godmother. "Do you want to understand more about what is going on with you and the relationship? I still have much to teach you."

"Yes, definitely!" exclaimed Cinderella, heartened by the prospect of further enlightenment.

"To begin with, let's talk about your emotional state," began Fairy Godmother. "As you allow your feelings of depression to lift, many unresolved and negative feelings from the past will bubble to the surface of your awareness. I urge you to recognize these feelings, cry about them and release them."

Fairy Godmother caught Cinderella's gaze and held it for several seconds before continuing, "I want to reassure you right now that you are completely okay. At times during the healing process you may feel like you're going crazy, but nothing could be further from the truth. Allowing the unconscious mind to bring forward past unresolved feelings, memories, thoughts and experiences is extremely valuable, even when it causes momentary distress and disorientation. It is also natural to have joyful feelings one minute as you carve out a bit more self-understanding, and be crying the next because you remember some past emotional injury."

A wave of trust softened Cinderella's eyes as she listened. Her gentle guardian truly understood the see-saw of emotions she was feeling.

"Whenever you bring forward emotional pain during our conversations, I will stop teaching and simply listen to you," promised Fairy Godmother. "Between sessions, when you feel upset, angry, sad or confused, just go with the experience. Write your reactions, thoughts and feelings in your journal — that will help you get through the experience. If you are busy with Marc and Mandy, wait until after their bedtime and then write — or steal a few moments while they are playing with Charming. Sometimes troubling emotions surface at inopportune times, but there are effective ways of managing such moments. For example, if you start feeling sad in the middle of a social event, you can say to yourself, 'I'll pay attention to my sadness this evening or tomorrow when I'm alone.' This technique can help you handle the demands of daily life. When public duties call, tell yourself to put all difficult emotions on hold. Your subconscious mind will obey you, *if* it has learned that you will express your unresolved feelings and write in your journal at a later time. If you renege on this agreement, you may find yourself crying at inconvenient times, unable to delay working with the feelings. So be good to yourself. Spend the necessary time so that you can heal," cautioned Fairy Godmother.

Cinderella took a deep breath and said, "I will do that. How long do you think all this emotional healing will take, a couple more months?"

Fairy Godmother smiled ruefully. "There you go again, trying to negotiate a crash course. This process takes as long as it takes. Place no judgments on the speed of your healing. Some people accomplish it in a year or two, others need a lifetime."

"Well, I certainly can't be doing this for years and years," replied Cinderella impatiently.

"Just know that I will be here to love and guide you for as long as you need me," soothed Fairy Godmother, ignoring Cinderella's restless eagerness. "So let's get back to learning more about marriage and relationships, shall we?"

"Yes, let's. I am ready for more of your teachings."

For a few moments Fairy Godmother closed her eyes in contemplation before resuming her lesson from the previous meeting. "Remember, Cindy, marriage is a perfect place to grow in consciousness. It provides the conditions necessary to expand self-awareness and progress on your spiritual journey. In marriage, you automatically have a mirror that shows you traits and qualities that you don't want to see in yourself. Most humans don't realize that they protect themselves by projecting onto others the parts of themselves which they can't own and accept. One way to recognize unconscious aspects of your personality is to watch yourself watching others. Notice what causes you to react, both positively and negatively. You can't recognize something in another person unless it already exists to some degree in you. Consider, for example, Charming's perception that you need too much attention. My guess is he would like a little more attention himself. But since he doesn't value emotional awareness, he is unable to acknowledge any feelings of neediness and wanting to be nurtured and cared for — needs that all humans occasionally experience, I might add. Long ago, as a young boy, Charming decided that the price of becoming emotionally dependent was too great to pay. Remember the smother love his mother gave him?"

"Yes, we discussed the part about his mother," said Cinderella. "And you're saying that he finds it easier to recognize and criticize my need for attention rather than deal with his own."

Fairy Godmother nodded emphatically. "He projects neediness onto you, disowning that part of himself. He judges that being needy is a bad trait, and so does his best to hide it from himself.

"The irony is that the things people despise and denounce in others are really the parts of themselves that they dislike, deny or fear," Fairy Godmother said with compassionate authority. "Mind you, such things are often not easy to see. The truth, as we've seen, has a way of sometimes revealing itself in opposites and symbols.

Take you for example. Why do you get so upset when Charming spends time enjoying himself out in the world?"

Cinderella sighed grimly, "Because he's not spending time with me."

"That's only part of it, my dear. Go deeper and see what else is inside."

Cinderella was quiet for several minutes before responding slowly, "I think that at some deep level, I wish that I too had meaningful work. Perhaps I'm bored with the roles I've accepted. Looking pretty and making sure the castle is in perfect order occupy time but aren't particularly challenging. I'd like to do something creative beyond my role as mother, wife and castle manager."

Cinderella looked a little doubtful, so Fairy Godmother jumped in. "That was excellent. As you get to know yourself more completely, you *will* discover creative urges and abilities that want to emerge and find expression. By responding to those urges, you will begin to develop valuable and rewarding pursuits of your own. And when you are busy with meaningful work, you won't pay much attention to what the prince is doing until the times when the two of you get together. On those occasions the excitement generated by your respective creative endeavors will give you much to share."

"But I don't want to sacrifice what little time I have with Charming. The good moments are so few and far between. If I'm busy, I'll see him even less," worried Cinderella, her eyebrows knotted with concern.

"You're right, physical meetings may at times take place less often than they do right now. I think you'll find that is okay, because the times you do have together will be of a much higher quality. They will not be based solely on romantic fulfillment as they were in the first stage of the relationship, nor will they be spent bickering, as they are now in the second stage. You'll have much to talk about because you'll both have new experiences to share," explained Fairy Godmother.

Cinderella was on her feet again, slowly circling the table. She listened intently as Fairy Godmother continued. "Add a close friend to your life, one who has interests and awareness similar to your own, and you'll forget to feel depressed and disappointed when Charming isn't particularly interested in listening to the details of your life. The prince will be happier, too, because he won't have to hear an elaborate account of each day's small events. When Charming is released from having to meet this need of yours, the relationship will be less stressed."

"When I'm honest with myself, I do think that some of my need for attention is really a manifestation of boredom. If I were busier with friends or activities of my own, like you're suggesting, I'd probably be easier to live with," said Cinderella. "And if that's true, then I'm probably projecting other things onto my husband, too."

"Yes," smiled Fairy Godmother, "I was just getting to that. The other day I asked you to spend some time writing down the things you like and dislike about Prince Charming. If you use your understanding of mirrors and projection, it will help you to clarify how these lists describe *you* as well as the prince."

"Aha! You had an ulterior motive for giving me that assignment," accused Cinderella, with mock indignation.

"Partly, yes. But I didn't conceal it for long. And I think you'll find that this process helps you to grow in awareness," said Fairy Godmother. "Parts of yourself that are disowned or denied have been projected onto Charming. Make some corrections in yourself and I guarantee you will see him differently. He may change, but even if he doesn't you will no longer be triggered by the things that bother you now."

Fairy Godmother clarified further. "This process can help you understand, heal and integrate experiences from early childhood as well. What you found difficult to understand or handle as a child is recreated in the present with Charming. Unconsciously, people find partners with some of the traits of their parents or caregivers. The negative traits you observe in Charming are clues to the areas where there is a need for new dance steps and new patterns of thinking and behaving. Remember, one of your childhood themes is not being cared for emotionally. That theme is reinforced each time Charming pulls away from you emotionally. Over time, *you* will be able to empower yourself, build your own self-esteem, and nurture the parts of yourself that were wounded in childhood. If Charming realizes that he, too, has much healing to accomplish, the scenario gets even better. Once in touch with his inner needs and conflicts and able to nurture himself, he'll more easily recognize when *you* need nurturing."

"That would be a dream come true," said Cinderella. Then, shaking her head, "It's kind of shocking to learn that one's parents have such a strong influence on the choice of a marriage partner and the dynamics of the relationship. I bet even step-parents are influential."

Fairy Godmother nodded and continued, "Marriage is a perfect place to balance inner polarities or conflicting attributes. People don't often see these inner conflicts until their partner acts out the opposing role. This signals the need to carve out a middle path between the two extremes. For example, when a wife gets angry a lot, her husband may develop the habit of remaining silent during confrontations or disagreements. Over time the quiet husband may have to face his own anger and not let the wife carry and express anger for both of them. The middle ground would necessitate the quiet husband learning to express anger when appropriate, and the angry wife learning to lighten up a bit. Another common example involves neatness versus sloppiness. Here it's easy to see how compromise could help restore balance to the relationship."

Cinderella laughed. "That sounds familiar. Charming isn't the least bit concerned where he throws his dirty clothes at night and many times they end up in the middle of the bedroom floor. I, on the other hand, can't stand having things out of place. We could both benefit from finding a happy medium."

"Yes, exactly. You may want to write in your journal about how you became so neat and tidy, describing the different emotions that come up over this issue. You can learn some very good lessons by looking at the small stuff," explained Fairy Godmother.

"Can you give me another example — one that involves deeper issues?" Cinderella asked. "I understand, but I want to take the concept a little further."

"Of course," replied Fairy Godmother. "Let's take you and your father. Do you think that your father had the same kind of relationship with your stepmother that you had as a child?"

"Of course not. If he had, he couldn't possibly have stayed married to her," huffed Cinderella.

"Good! My point exactly. Your father was a good man and would never have left you in the care of an abusive woman if he had been able to recognize her cruel, vindictive nature. Why do you suppose he failed to see those qualities?" asked Fairy Godmother.

"Well, if I apply the concept of our being mirrors for each other and sometimes working through opposites, I have to conclude that he didn't suspect her negative intentions because he never had them himself," Cinderella replied. "And he traveled a great deal, so for the short periods that he was home, she managed to deceive him with a sweet facade. As soon as he left, the dam broke and she burst into one of her tirades."

Reflecting on her own words, Cinderella observed, "I must have some of my father's traits. Until you began explaining this to me, I never really saw her as abusive. I guess I was a little naive, too."

"Very good, Cindy!" replied Fairy Godmother, clapping loudly to acknowledge Cinderella for her developing insight.

The two companions continued to chat about areas of the marital relationship where Cinderella and Charming believed and behaved like polar opposites. They discussed ways of resolving these conflicts and achieving more balance. As their discussion wound down, Cinderella's demeanor became increasingly serious. Finally she said, "A while ago you mentioned enthusiasm and depression as being polarities, probably because you see them in us. I recognize them, too. But the interesting thing is, we seem to be reversing roles. As I've become happier, a cloud has formed over Charming's head. I guess we both have each of these traits."

"Yes, that's an excellent observation, Cindy," said Fairy Godmother without further comment.

"I need time to internalize all this information," said Cinderella, "but I like the idea of concentrating more on myself and not constantly focusing on my partner. After all, my task is to understand me."

"Yes," said Fairy Godmother with obvious pleasure. "The focus is on you, not Prince Charming."

"What questions do you have for me to answer in my journal today?" asked Cinderella.

"I want you to explore the mirror and polarity concepts in writing, and apply them to yourself and the relationship," replied Fairy Godmother, producing a sheet of paper. Here, these should get you started."

Cinderella accepted the list and quickly scanned the questions. When she looked up, her guardian had vanished.

1. Write (but don't send) a letter to anyone who wounded you in the past.

2. By noticing things you admire and dislike in your partner, write about your unconscious or shadow side. Use the mirror concept.

3. List polarities that you and your partner act out in your relationship; for example, enthusiasm versus depression. Explore in writing those that bother you, and describe any insights you develop.

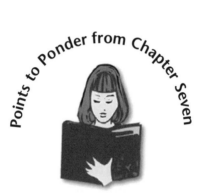

Points to Ponder from Chapter Seven

1. When challenged in a relationship, look at the big picture to see life lessons that will help expedite the change process.

2. Letting emotional pain surface is healthy and facilitates healing.

3. Learn about yourself by examining the projections that you have placed on others and that they have mirrored back to you.

    Sometimes projections are mirror images of your behaviors, traits, patterns or beliefs, and sometimes they take the form of polarities — reflecting your exact opposite. Polarities may also exist within you. Balancing and integrating these polarities speeds your journey to wholeness.

4. Understanding the mirror concept can help you to heal and integrate experiences from early childhood, and not project them onto your partner.

Polarities in the relationship help pinpoint areas where self-understanding and growth are needed. Your partner mirrors your blind spots. Instead of wishing that your partner were different, redirect the energy on your own behalf. Claim the parts that you have projected.

5. When you react negatively to your partner, examine yourself in relation to the trigger issue.

    Identify what in you needs healing relative to the issue. Rather than continue to project outside of yourself, decide to own what you see.

6. When you own what you like and dislike in your partner, the projections are removed.

    Your partner no longer has to act them out for you. You are really a whole person in your own right, and so is your partner. You both deserve to know the real person behind the projections. Even if you understand and practice this and your partner still projects, your awareness will enable you to communicate differently, explaining what you see.

7. In a healthy relationship, each partner is encouraged to manifest his/her true self.

    A bridge of understanding is built from soul to soul, moving the couple beyond dramas and negative patterns. Partners take responsibility to heal their own part of the dance.

8. The healing process is aided by writing (but not mailing) letters to people who have hurt you in the past.

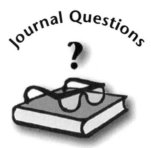

Journal Questions ?

For greater introspection, answer the questions about mirrors and polarities that Fairy Godmother gave to Cinderella.

Chapter Eight

Cinderella Expresses Much Pain

"Good morning, Godmother," Cinderella called through the open glass doors connecting her private sitting room to the garden alcove. "I'll be right there."

Fairy Godmother was already waiting beside the alcove table. "Isn't it a glorious day?" she called back, stretching her arms out to envelop the midmorning sun. A moment later Cinderella joined her. As they hugged, a chorus of birds could be heard singing in the nearby orchard.

Cinderella and her guardian had been meeting for over a month, but this encounter was destined to be a little different. Through reading and journal writing, the princess had been reaching deeper and deeper levels of awareness. Many were proving too painful to manage alone.

"The day may be glorious, but I'm not," sighed Cinderella as she dropped listlessly into a chair. "Charming is rejecting me again. When I approach him, he stiffens and I can tell he doesn't want me to touch him. And he certainly doesn't touch me! The emotional distance between us seems to have widened since I started talking to you. I want so much to have a warm, loving relationship like we had in the beginning. I want to begin relating on a soul level and don't know how. When I try to talk about how I feel, he listens for a minute and then interrupts with some silly, irrelevant question like, 'What are the kids going to wear to the tournament next Saturday?' Or he stares at me stone-faced and makes no response at all — or looks right past me, daydreaming. The less he responds, the harder I try to reach him. Invariably I begin to cry, to which he grumbles, 'Not this again!'"

Cinderella continued, "It seems that the more I try to express how I feel, the more intense I get and the further he retreats. It doesn't help to be silent, either. He avoids me. *Either way* he avoids me. I feel so empty and unloved. How can this be happening to me? I'm afraid he doesn't want to be with me." Cinderella's sighs turned to sobs. Fairy Godmother sat quietly, producing an endless supply of handkerchiefs.

"Last night in bed we didn't touch all night," mumbled Cinderella through the soaked cloth. "Usually we at least hug a little."

With this last revelation, Cinderella's crying became agonized. Her body shook as though emitting more pain than it had tears to ease. Her shoulders and arms were tight and tense, her anguish compounded by the growling, moaning, gut-wrenching sounds she produced. The poor creature — you'd have thought Charming was dead and her heart broken.

This whole transforming process was like a death experience. Fairy Godmother knew it, and had been waiting for the crash. When a person receives helpful, healing teachings, she wants to be able to put them into practice — to live them — not have her efforts thwarted at every turn. When Fairy Godmother talked about the healing process to Cinderella, she knew challenging times were ahead — times like today. In her wisdom, Fairy

Godmother didn't attempt to stifle Cinderella's tears, but instead sent her healing energy.

And then, just as suddenly as the tears and moaning had begun, they stopped. Cinderella, who had buried her face in Fairy Godmother's lap, sat up and haltingly resumed her story right where she had left off. "I wanted to make love last night and Charming refused me. He didn't say no in words, he simply didn't respond. He lay there motionless with his eyes closed until he fell asleep. He knows it's hard for me to ask. I feel embarrassed and humiliated. What do I do now? Why is this happening to me?" asked Cinderella. "I don't understand it at all."

Fairy Godmother just listened. She considered it unwise to give information or try to solve problems in the face of such emotion. Developing insight required a clear mind. For the moment, listening with a kind ear was enough.

Fairy Godmother did not agree with everything Cinderella had said. But agreement wasn't what Cinderella sought. She needed a good cry, so Fairy Godmother decided to save her interpretations until a better time.

Cinderella began to remember and describe other times she'd felt emotionally wounded in life. Every detail of the past seemed vivid. Many of the things she said about Charming were surprising. Some were harsh and difficult to believe. Others would not have bothered most women in Cinderella's place.

The safety of Fairy Godmother's presence kept Cinderella talking and eventually calmed her. A dozen or so small animals that had gathered during Cinderella's outburst now went about their business, scurrying from place to place while Cinderella and Fairy Godmother watched. The squirrels and rabbits were obviously sensitive to Cinderella's pain and willing to convey a heavy dose of unconditional love. Their effect was as healing as Fairy Godmother's.

At last Fairy Godmother spoke. "I think it best that we not discuss any new ideas today. You just purged yourself of a great deal of pent-up pain. It was very important work. Your body has been holding those feelings for a long, long time — especially the feelings of grief and abandonment from the early loss of your parents. I recommend that you sit here as usual and write for a while after I leave."

"Oh, please," cried Cinderella. "Just a few ideas to ponder. I need your guidance to help me interpret my emotions. I'm okay, really, just tired — and still hungry for your wisdom."

Fairy Godmother sat in silent deliberation for a few moments, weighing her options. She decided to plant a seed about the real search that Cinderella was engaged in — the spiritual quest.

Fairy Godmother explained that much of Cinderella's yearning for closeness with Charming was a yearning for God, a connection with her own soul, and a reunion with the spiritual world that at times was felt but not remembered.

"As you make it through these deep painful emotions, you will eventually be able to redirect your energies to connecting with your higher self, which some people call the soul and others call the *transpersonal* self. The first part of this spiritual journey involves knowing yourself and healing your consciousness, which you are already doing. Eventually, you will begin to remember who you really are. Much of your present identity — who you think and feel you are — is a result of your past experiences. Therefore, you must continue to gain a better understanding of the traumas, unresolved griefs, relationships with caregivers, and other elements of your childhood. You will continue to benefit by understanding how these experiences affect you in the present. Your inner child's interpretations of early experiences can make you feel like a victim in adulthood," explained Fairy Godmother.

After a quick assessment of Cinderella's emotional state, she decided to ignore her earlier statement about not discussing anything new today. "For example, when Charming didn't respond to you last night, you interpreted his behavior through the filter of past hurts, and you felt victimized. Because you felt rejected by your father, who had little time for you, the same feelings arose in response to Charming's disinterest. The prince probably wasn't out to hurt you at all. Perhaps he was tired. He may even have felt victimized — by you touching him when he needed space, or by the fact that you are changing."

"Are you serious?" asked Cinderella, incredulous. "I never thought that I might be abusing *him*."

"Well, I think 'victimize' and 'abuse' are probably too harsh for this situation, but pestering someone who wants to sleep is definitely an invasion of privacy. Your timing was off for sure. The more you and Charming understand your respective ways of responding to each other, the better you'll be able to choose behaviors that help both of you to grow out of the past," explained Fairy Godmother.

"Like what?" asked Cinderella with interest.

"Well, over time you may be able to teach Charming that if he holds you for a minute or two when he's not in the mood for lovemaking, you won't perceive his lack of interest as rejection," replied Fairy Godmother.

"You're right, that would help," exclaimed Cinderella. "Shall I tell him that? We have so many things that we don't talk about and..."

"Hold on, I'm not finished," cautioned Fairy Godmother. "Another solution is for you to change your interpretation of his coolness. Don't take everything so personally. Instead of seeing his lack of interest as rejection, learn to see it as a function of his present mood, and remind yourself that he may be in an entirely different mood tomorrow."

"That would not be so easy, but I do see your point."

"I want to back up a minute to your statement that there are many subjects about which you and Charming don't talk at all. If and when we engage Charming in inner healing work, this situation will change and the two of you will be able to discuss who's wounded inner child has the most urgent needs. If, on a particular night, you determine that Charming's need for space is greater than your need for closeness, then meeting his need will be best for the relationship at that time. On the other hand, if your need to talk about your feelings is greater than his need to be alone, then meeting your need will be best."

Cinderella stared at the table for a long time, tears welling up in her eyes. "Making decisions like that takes two very caring and mature people. I don't think we qualify."

"Yes, you're right," agreed Fairy Godmother. "It takes *two* people to create a good relationship. With only one person doing the work, the road is rough and very slow. One person can serve as the catalyst by bringing new information into the relationship, but eventually both partners must take responsibility."

"I don't know what to do next," complained Cinderella. "I'm stuck."

Fairy Godmother thought for a minute. "I think this is a good time for you to write a letter to Charming. And I think you need to give it to him. Express your concerns, your intentions, and be specific about the kind of relationship you want to have."

"How can I do that when I don't really know myself?" demanded Cinderella. "What if I express myself poorly? I don't have the right words."

"You don't have to write a perfect letter. What's important is making the effort to communicate with your husband. Look, here's some simple advice. Speak about your experience. Talk about what you think, feel and need. The best way to do this is with I-messages rather than you-messages. For example, it's better to say, 'I am upset,' than 'You make me upset'. This way you won't sound like you are preaching to or criticizing him."

"Yes, using I-messages is much more positive. I'm willing to write the letter, but I feel somewhat skeptical. You are absolutely right when you say all this awareness takes time to assimilate. I can hardly understand myself right now, let alone explain myself properly to Charming," admitted Cinderella.

"I have no doubt that you will write an effective letter. In fact, doing so will help you to clarify your thoughts, feelings and needs. I know you can do it," encouraged Fairy Godmother.

"Thank you. I'm so grateful that you are here to support me until I feel safe communicating on my own," said Cinderella.

"Would you like a meditation to help you build a bridge of communication with Charming — to set the stage, so to speak?"

"Most definitely," replied Cinderella.

"By using the power of visualization, you can direct energy to the creation of a new relationship that arises at the soul level — the kind of relationship we've been talking about. Remember, while you can achieve this connection in spirit, it won't fully manifest on a concrete level unless the prince is equally committed to it. When two people are involved, reality must be co-created. Forcing another to do anything is a misuse of power, even when it is clearly for the highest good. Free will and choice must always be respected," explained Fairy Godmother.

"Then why even do it?" questioned Cinderella.

"Because by visualizing, you actually *see* the higher path that is *your* goal, and seeing the image facilitates the process. Eventually, you will create this kind of relationship for yourself even if the prince is unable or unwilling to join you. If and when he does join you, the process will work much faster because it will have been preceded by much inner work on your part. And if he *never* comes around, you'll eventually create the relationship with someone better suited to you."

"I don't want to think about that. I only want this with Charming," objected Cinderella.

"I know, dear, and we won't jump to possible futures unless one lands in your lap. Right now let me guide you on this meditation," said Fairy Godmother.

"Okay, that's fair."

After making sure they were in a secluded part of the garden, Fairy Godmother began speaking to Cinderella slowly in a low voice. "Close your eyes and take some deep breaths... As you inhale, breathe in love and peace and calmness... As you exhale, let go of tension, fear and tightness... Go to your place of peace. This can be a place you imagine or one you've actually visited. If you are not a visual person, try to experience feelings and sensations... Feel golden white light shining on the top of your head, filling you up with healing energy. The excess flows from your hands and feet and enters the earth, where it is used as the planet sees fit... Now, invite Charming into your place of peace... See him radiant... He too is filled with this golden white light... Imagine a bridge between the two of you. You walk toward each other from opposite sides of the bridge... Your faces are aglow with love... Begin talking to the prince. Tell him how you love him. Describe to him the relationship you want to create. Be specific... Listen to and hear whatever he has to say."

Fairy Godmother paused for a minute or two and then continued.

"Now, it is time to release Charming and return to the garden. Visualize the two of you kissing and embracing, then walking back to opposite ends of the bridge. Come back to your place of peace feeling rested. Become aware of your body. Now, bring your awareness back to the garden, slowly open your eyes and begin moving and stretching."

Cinderella was quiet for a few minutes. Rubbing her eyes, she said in a calm voice, "That was wonderful. I feel much better."

"I think we've done enough for today. Just sit quietly in the garden, dear," suggested Fairy Godmother. "This is a perfect time to allow your unconscious to bring up any issues that stand in the way of building a good relationship with Charming. As you know, sometimes roadblocks arise from past events or relationships that seem to have nothing to do with the present situation. Just be open for a few minutes while you sit here alone in your garden."

Once she was sure Cinderella understood her directions, Fairy Godmother said good-bye and disappeared.

Cinderella sat for a long while. In her quietude, a small, silent voice within told her to express her feelings in letters to her stepmother and stepsisters — letters that would remain in her journal and contribute to her healing. Cinderella could see that in order to create the highest relationship with the prince, she needed to confront some of the wounds she'd experienced at the hands of these women. Making peace with them was very important to her healing. To Cinderella's surprise, she easily recorded exactly what she was thinking and feeling. The process of writing released much pain.

Cinderella then began a letter to Charming. This one would be delivered.

Dear Charming:

There is much I want to say, but lately I don't know how to talk to you. I have been in a great deal of pain without even realizing it. It seems that you do not want to be around me at times and this has caused my mind to create many unhappy scenarios. I really do not know what is true anymore. I feel rejected and depressed. For a while I thought you were rejecting me because I didn't want to compete with you in the tournaments. Then I thought you might be reacting to my low moods. But over the past few days I've been extremely happy at times and this, too, seems to put you off.

I don't feel close to you anymore, and I can't seem to talk to you. I miss both. So much has been happening inside me lately and I would love to share these things with you. I know that I ramble when I talk. You've often commented that I never get to the point. But, I really have figured out a lot about me, about you, and about us. For example, I now realize that many of my expectations about our relationship have been idealistic. The time has come to be realistic.

I am crying as I write this. Maybe I need to write to you more often. If you could read my ideas on paper, you wouldn't have to feel uncomfortable and irritated that I can't say anything once I start crying.

Oh, I love you so much. I want more than anything to spend some time with you. Can we meet in the garden tonight when the children are in bed?

Love,

Cindy

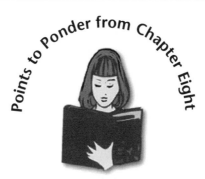

Points to Ponder from Chapter Eight

1. Putting new ideas into practice takes time.

    Behaving in accordance with concepts you have learned and
    accepted intellectually can be a slow and frustrating process.
    Trust that you are progressing at your own perfect pace. Use
    self-help books and guided meditations to promote
    understanding and healing.

2. Allowing painful feelings to surface is an important part of
    healing.

    The term breakdown is descriptive of the process. Old patterns,
    behaviors and beliefs are "breaking down" because they are no
    longer working. Deep-felt crying accompanied by intense sound-
    making helps eliminate pain from the body.

3. When the pain of understanding and change gets too intense to
    bear alone, arrange to be with a trusted friend, counselor or
    spiritual helper.

4. In reality, Cinderella's search is a spiritual quest.

    Longing for closeness and wanting a partner to be there for you
    symbolize a desire to be close to God or one's higher self. The
    beginning of this spiritual journey is to know yourself inside and
    out.

5. Many partner conflicts are played out between each one's
    wounded inner child.

To change the pattern and open up communication, attempt to communicate from your adult state.

6. The victim-victimizer pattern changes between partners.

   When you don't know your effect on your partner, you can mistakenly victimize him.

7. If you have difficulty talking to your partner, write and deliver a letter that states your feelings and needs and addresses problematic issues in the relationship.

   Speak from experience and use I-messages.

8. One person can improve a relationship; two are required to create a good relationship.

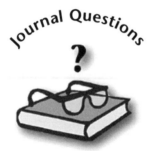

Journal Questions

?

Write a letter to your partner expressing your deepest thoughts and feelings.

Chapter Nine

Working Together

The next time Fairy Godmother appeared in the garden, she was startled to see Charming sitting next to Cinderella at the alcove table. "Well, what a nice surprise!" she said, smiling at the two of them.

"I wrote to Charming after our last meeting, and he responded by joining us today," explained Cinderella. "I was happy to learn that he, too, has been concerned about our relationship. We talked for a long time and I feel a lot better."

"That's good news. Talking and listening help most situations," responded Fairy Godmother. "Where would you like to begin today?"

"I want Charming to hear some of the things we've been talking about concerning relationships and personal growth. I think it will help him to understand me better. I want him to realize why we haven't been getting along lately, why we're together, and how to improve our communication when we don't understand each other," said Cinderella eagerly.

Fairy Godmother noticed at once that Charming looked uncomfortable and needed to be brought into the conversation. "And you, Charming, why are you here today? And what do you hope to receive from this meeting?" she asked.

"Well, I'm not really sure," Charming responded guardedly. "I do care about Cindy and our relationship, even though she hasn't thought so lately, and I decided it might be a good idea to come and observe today. Perhaps if I watch for a little while I'll begin to understand why she's in such a whirlwind about you. I don't really think we have much of a problem, but Cindy has been acting so strangely lately that I'm confused. Her intensity is overwhelming, to say the least."

"Thank you, it helps to know your thoughts," nodded Fairy Godmother. "I can imagine that the relationship is a challenge for you right now. And talking to Cindy probably creates even more confusion. She is learning new concepts and doesn't yet understand everything we've discussed. In fact, I'll bet that while attempting to describe these new concepts, not fully understanding them herself, she skips vital information and can't defend her positions."

"Yes, that must be what's going on," said Charming. "When I ask questions or want more information, Cindy just gets irritated with me and accuses me of not listening, doubting her word, or starts crying. So I actually find it easier to avoid her."

"Godmother, please explain to him some of the ideas so he can understand them better," Cinderella urged.

Fairy Godmother smiled patiently. "All of that information will emerge in it's own time," she said gently, "if not directly from me, then when the two of you are talking. Rather than teach Charming anything, Cindy, I'd rather we just talk. All the ideas will surface at the appropriate time. I encourage both of you to realize that your relationship is in a volatile state. Things will feel unstable and confusing much of the time, so you need to talk whenever possible. But don't force it."

"I'm not sure we know how to talk without getting into an argument," sighed Cinderella. "I begin talking and Charming just does not understand what I'm saying. If he asks a question that I can't answer, I get frustrated and angry. Then he says something that hurts my feelings — usually having to do with the children. He implies that I'm doing something wrong."

"That's not true, Cindy," interjected Charming.

"Yes it is. Last night when I was explaining that I needed to be more independent, you interrupted when you heard Marc crying outside. You said that he wouldn't cry so much if I hadn't been so soft on him when he was little," accused Cinderella.

"But that's because he's got to be king someday and..."

"There you go again, blaming me because Marc isn't tough emotionally like you are," said Cinderella.

The prince closed his eyes and shook his head in weary frustration. Fairy Godmother waited patiently for the two of them to settle down, watching all the time as Cinderella attempted to describe her feelings or perceptions and Charming interrupted defensively. Each expressed a different interpretation of almost everything, reacted emotionally, and both talked at the same time.

"Stop!" Fairy Godmother said finally. "Both of you are entirely correct from your point of view, but being right doesn't help a relationship very much. From now on, I'm going to ask that we all adhere to a set of simple communication rules. And I'd like you to follow the same rules when I'm not around. They will help you begin to settle your differences. She handed them each a copy of the following rules and suggested that they take it in turns to read them aloud.

Opening Communication:
Guidelines for Resolving Conflict and Fighting Fairly

1. **Stick to the subject.** Discuss one topic at a time. Do not confuse issues. If your partner attempts to change the subject, simply say, "That's important, but let's finish this first." Completing discussions produces feelings of satisfaction and closure.

2. **Deal with feelings.** If your partner is emotional, wait while the feelings are expressed. Effective communication gets to the bottom of issues that may look insignificant or even silly on the surface. If your partner gets extremely emotional, recognize that his/her actions are a clue that something is going on beneath the surface. Help your partner by asking questions like, "What are you feeling?" If your partner is unable to identify the feelings, offer a little help. Anger, for example, indicates the presence of some other primary emotion, like shame, embarrassment, fear, rejection, abandonment, or feeling "taken advantage of."

3. **Take turns listening and expressing.** Good communication requires that partners express themselves honestly and accurately while paying attention to what the other partner is saying. Both persons must assume both roles at different times.

4. **Stay in the present.** Express what you are thinking and feeling right now, even if the event you are talking about happened in the past or will take place in the future.

5. **Speak from your own experience.** No two people experience an incident the same way. Do not expect your partner to know what you think and feel. You are unique.

You have your own history, conditioning, perceptions and beliefs. Take responsibility for yourself by using statements such as, "I believe...," "As I see it...," "I feel...," "In my opinion...," "I experience...," "I am aware..."

6. **Use empathic, active listening.** Listen between the lines and look for meaning beyond the spoken words. When your partner is talking, show caring and respect by making eye contact, facing your partner, nodding your head or saying things like, "Yes, I understand," "Tell me more," or "I don't understand." Use a supportive tone of voice. Do not interrupt.

7. **Attack the problem, not the person.** Avoid unkind personal comments, criticisms and name calling. Agreeing with everything your partner says is not necessary, but hearing all sides of an issue is. Always honor your partner, even when you don't like what s/he says or does.

8. **Find win-win solutions.** After you and your partner have thoroughly discussed an issue, take time to look for creative solutions that are agreeable to both of you. Compromise is necessary sometimes. Honor your partner and do not attempt to dominate the solution process.

"Whew," breathed Charming, putting down his list. "Remembering all this is going to be tough. Don't get me wrong, I think the rules are good. But the idea of having to frame every thought according to a set of guidelines strikes me as pretty restrictive."

"The rules may be difficult to follow at first," acknowledged Fairy Godmother, "but I can promise you that they are far less encumbering than the anger and defensiveness generated by poor communication. They will help you to listen without reacting, to hear each other's ideas in an atmosphere of mutual respect. Confrontation is good if you fight fairly; however, when you hear only part of what the other person says, your emotions are triggered by unfinished business from the past and nothing gets resolved. Just as you learn to frame every move in a joust according to the tournament rules, you will grow accustomed to these rules with practice. It may take a little time, but it is well worth it and will serve you in the long run."

"I think we should give the rules a try," interjected Cinderella earnestly, reaching out to touch Charming's arm. "They are bound to help us."

"Okay, I'll do my best, Cindy, but you will probably have to remind me sometimes."

Charming turned his attention to Fairy Godmother. "A moment ago, you mentioned that feelings can be triggered by unfinished business from the past. What type of 'unfinished business'?" he inquired.

Cinderella sat very quietly as Fairy Godmother and Charming discussed how the past affects the present. Fairy Godmother explained many ideas that the princess had already heard. For example, she talked about the need to update perceptions and to identify guiding beliefs. And she explained that when one partner has an overly emotional reaction it usually means that previous experiences are leaking into and affecting the present response.

"Whatever is happening in the current moment reminds you at an unconscious level of an earlier negative experience and the feelings associated with it. So you automatically react defensively in the new situation. You get that ancient 'fight or flight' stress response where chemicals from the brain pour into the bloodstream to give you a burst of energy. The energy is so intense that you react out of proportion to the situation. The bigger the reaction, the bigger the need to identify the past experiences that are leaking into the present. Only by understanding them can you transform the situation," explained Fairy Godmother.

The trio talked at length about many topics — how one's family of origin affects the current relationship, and even the stages a couple go through in a relationship.

"Some of this is starting to make sense to me now," said the prince during a lull in the discussion. "I'm not sure I agree with everything — and don't know what I need to do with this information — but I definitely understand better where Cindy is coming from. I am more receptive to using these ideas — even the communication guidelines — to improve our relationship."

"That's a relief," sighed Cinderella.

"There, you see?" smiled Fairy Godmother, getting up from the table. Understanding, even without agreement, builds trust and openness." She gazed up at the late afternoon sky, which was starting to cloud up. "It's getting late, and I must take my leave. Keep those communication guidelines handy and let me know how it goes," she called cheerfully as she dematerialized.

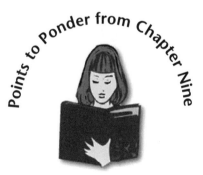

Points to Ponder from Chapter Nine

1. When one partner gathers information about relationships and personal growth while the other does little or nothing, the effect is usually unsettling.

The person gathering the information is likely to get a little too pushy, which causes the partner to feel threatened, confused or fearful. The partner's response is often to withdraw and avoid talking. All of this is normal behavior.

2. Everyone gathers and assimilates new information at a different pace.

    Factors influencing the rate of assimilation include one's interest, experience and ability. Usually partners do not match in these areas. It helps to understand each other's pace.

3. Unfinished business from the past often causes emotional reactions greater than the current situation warrants.

4. You are 100 percent correct from your point of view — and so is your partner.

    However, being right does not solve relationship problems.

5. Whenever possible it is good to bring both partners together for relationship counseling.

    The process of counseling creates common experiences and common ground on which to discuss problems and take shared responsibility for building a better relationship.

6. Confrontation is good if ground rules are established.

7. Specific, tangible communication techniques and skills can be learned and practiced.

    Understanding and listening to a partner's point of view builds trust and understanding. Agreement is not the goal.

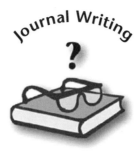

Journal Writing

?

As you go about your day, recall the communication guidelines that Fairy Godmother gave to Cinderella and Charming. Attempt to put them into practice. If your partner is willing, share the guidelines and see what discussion follows. If your partner is unwilling, you will have to move a little more slowly. In either case, remember to record insights and process your feelings in your journal. This will help you to clarify your thinking and to communicate more clearly and easily.

Now we are ready to end the story of Cinderella and Prince Charming. Because life is unpredictable when two people co-create a relationship, the story has two possible endings. Most people want a happy ending — one in which the partners stay together. But not staying together needn't automatically lead to an unhappy ending. The high divorce rate in Western society suggests that many couples would benefit by learning to end their relationships on a positive note before moving on to a better life. Both conclusions — staying together and splitting apart — represent valid outcomes.

Chapter Ten

Ending Number One
The Completion

The lessons with Fairy Godmother continued for many months. Cinderella, by now an avid student, met with her loving teacher often. The two spent hours discussing various ideas and insights. Charming found time to accompany Cinderella about once or twice a month. He grew to enjoy these encounters with Fairy Godmother and clearly desired to know himself better and work on his relationship with Cinderella.

Cinderella and the prince were sitting silently on opposite sides of the alcove table when Fairy Godmother appeared on this warm day in early June, fourteen months after her first visit. She observed the two shrewdly while winding her way to the table through lush tiers of flowering sage. "It appears that you two have something to tell me," she observed, brushing purple petals from her skirt and taking a chair between them.

"Yes," replied Cinderella. "We've been up all night talking. Though this process hasn't been easy, it has forced us to look at why we are together. Some of the reasons are not too healthy.

Much to my dismay, we've made a decision I thought I'd never agree to. We've come to the conclusion that we need to separate. I feel sad and relieved at the same time, which is quite confusing."

Fairy Godmother noticed tears in both pairs of tired eyes. "I want to hear more about your decision" she said. "but first tell me about your sadness. You first, Cindy."

"I hurt deep inside, like a piece has been ripped out of my stomach. I've been weeping for hours and I'm exhausted. Even though I'm certain we've made the right decision, I feel like I'm leaving my best friend, my roots, my security."

Choking up a bit, she stammered, "I know it's the right thing to do, but I can't believe it's turning out this way. I thought that all our relationship needed was for Charming to understand the information you were teaching me about relationships — about becoming your own authority, building self-esteem and understanding how your family of origin affects you as an adult."

The prince interjected, "But it didn't work that way. The more I found out about who I really am, the more I had to admit that I'm not suited to this marriage — perhaps not to any marriage. I became a husband for the wrong reasons. My family was pressuring me to produce an heir. Almost nothing was said about compatibility, goals, values and beliefs. Cindy and I are growing and changing so fast that we have little in common anymore, so little in fact that the strong attraction we experienced in the beginning of the relationship is gone."

Cinderella continued, "I assumed that in getting to know ourselves we would automatically find reasons to stay together. It's so sad."

Charming put his hand on Cinderella's shoulder and patiently waited for her to calm down. His eyes were soft with empathy. "I want to separate more than Cindy does. She can make the best of any situation, and would stay in an unhappy marriage forever.

When we began these sessions last year, I wasn't aware that deep down inside I really wanted out of the relationship. It sounds a little cold, but I'm fairly certain that I don't want to be married. I'm a loner. The need to constantly relate is an unwelcome intrusion. I don't like to admit these thoughts and feelings because I don't enjoy causing Cindy so much pain. Nevertheless, they're true."

"I admire your willingness to be clear and honest. How long have you known?" asked Fairy Godmother.

"He's known for a long time, maybe a couple of months," Cinderella answered, wiping her eyes. "He told me about a week ago, right after our last meeting with you. At first, I just wanted to be alone. That's why you haven't seen me in the garden this week. I'm still crying a lot, but I'm starting to come to terms with the reality of the situation."

"Don't rush it, Cinderella. You're in a grieving process. Working through your sadness could easily take a year or two. And you'll need a lot of emotional support," Fairy Godmother said gently.

"Can you explain what you mean by 'grieving process'?" requested the prince.

Nodding, Fairy Godmother continued, "Grieving over a separation or divorce is similar to grieving over the death of a loved one. At first you are in a state of shock, unable to believe what is happening. You say things like, 'Why me?' and 'This can't be true,' while denying the reality of the situation. At the moment, I see Cindy expressing some of these things. I'm not sure about you, Charming."

Fairy Godmother resumed her explanation. "In most cases, shock and disbelief soon change to anger. You may want to blame the other person or strike out in some way. Next, you may experience glimmers of hope and try to bargain with yourselves, with each other or with God by promising to do things differently in exchange for saving the marriage. When you realize that you can't control the situation, you will probably feel frustrated, which may lead to a desire to isolate yourself. Depression usually follows and is a normal reaction. Eventually you will come to terms with the reality of the situation and accept the death of the marriage. Most people cycle through these stages over and over, experiencing a tumult of emotions for quite some time — long after they've understood and accepted the situation. Birthdays, holidays and anniversaries are especially apt to generate renewed grieving."

"I must be in shock," said Charming, "because I feel numb. Even though I'm the one pushing to separate, the reality of it is still frightening. I didn't plan it."

"I understand," said Fairy Godmother. "Even the person asking for the separation and divorce goes through the same grieving process."

The three of them sat very still for several minutes. Finally, Fairy Godmother broke the silence. "Have you discussed the details?" she asked.

"Some of them," answered Charming. "Cindy will probably move into town. She will have the children for the majority of the time because that's what they're accustomed to and because she loves her role as a mother. I'll support her until such time as she chooses to remarry."

"If I ever do," interrupted Cinderella, with an angry edge.

Looking a little chagrined, Charming continued, "Marc will travel back and forth fairly often between the city and the castle so that he may continue preparing for the day when he will assume the throne. My tutors and mentors are working with him already. I will always make time for Marc and Mandy. Cinderella and I agree that they need both of us."

"The hardest part will be telling everyone," worried Cinderella. "We lead such a charmed life, people assume we must be happy. How I dread facing my two stepsisters. I feel like such a failure."

"There's another way to look at divorce," responded Fairy Godmother encouragingly. She proceeded to explain her views on mistakes and failure. "Divorce can be seen as a creative experience with conscious choices. Instead of viewing the marriage as a mistake, see it as the best choice available to you at the time, given what you knew about yourselves. The fact that you would do things differently if you could go back in time today, with your current level of awareness, does not mean that you chose poorly at the time. Ten years ago you didn't know yourselves or your choices very well. Remember that life is a creative experience. Look at all you have experienced and learned from the union and vow to go forward from this day considering your choices carefully. Take lots of time when making long range decisions, like choosing a life partner. Listen to your intuition and inner self."

Cinderella smiled ruefully. "I will certainly ask for your guidance if there is a next time."

"I hope that by then you will know yourself so well that you won't need me. You will be able to act on your own inner guidance. Of course, I will always be available to talk," reassured Fairy Godmother lovingly.

"Thank you," returned Cinderella.

"I think it would be a good idea to continue our joint sessions for a while," urged Fairy Godmother. "You two may need the help of an objective party when dealing with some of the emotional issues ahead."

"That sounds okay to me," said Charming.

"Me too," said Cinderella.

128

The three of them talked for most of the afternoon. They discussed how to tell Marc and Mandy and how to make the transition easier for them. Fairy Godmother created a safe place for both Cinderella and Charming to share their deepest feelings honestly and openly. The two talked about the good times and expressed appreciation for the many gifts of learning and experience they had given each other. And they pledged to be mature enough to work together productively as parents. When the session was over, an aura of peace and completion settled over the garden.

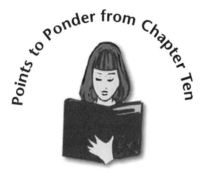

Points to Ponder from Chapter Ten

1. Couples need to look at why they are together.

    Shared interests, goals and purpose are necessary to maintain a partnership. Relationships are co-created. A good task for couples is periodically to talk about what they have in common and where they are headed. An occasional reality check avoids surprises and discourages wishful thinking.

2. Couples can benefit from meeting with a therapist, counselor, or teacher to facilitate growth, both individually and in the marriage.

    A person whose frame of reference is both professional and objective can guide partners to greater awareness and help them to see new possibilities. However, counseling and good communication do not ensure that a marriage will stay together.

3. Joint counseling opens communication and helps couples find solutions to their problems.

    Should a couple choose to separate, divorce counseling can facilitate a smooth transition.

4. A divorce is like a death, and produces a similar grieving process.

5. Divorce does not equal failure, and can be used as a creative experience.

6. A good divorce bases choices on the best interests of each family member, especially the children.

Chapter Eleven

Ending Number Two
The Magic of Transformation

Charming's initial lesson in the garden turned out to be the first of many. He grew to enjoy his encounters with Fairy Godmother and he made up his mind that he wanted to know himself better and to work on his relationship with Cinderella.

Cinderella and Charming learned that the ups and downs of daily living were easier to navigate when a strong relationship nurtured and supported their individual journeys. They learned to communicate more effectively and to understand patterns of behavior from their respective pasts that needed healing. When either of them had an "off" day, the other attempted to provide support by recalling appropriate lessons from Fairy Godmother's garden classroom. They learned to be open, to share feelings, and to resolve personal, relationship and family issues through joint problem solving. With honesty and caring, they set about building an emotionally close relationship in which intimacy grew daily.

On an afternoon in late October, a couple of years after their first meeting with her, Cinderella and Charming discussed their relationship with Fairy Godmother.

"It's not that we do everything perfectly, or always agree, or never try to control each other," stated Charming. "But when we have problems, we're able to work them out because our relationship has a strong foundation now."

"I agree," said Cinderella. "What Charming and I have is very different from what I envisioned the first few times I met with you, Fairy Godmother. The relationship is a lot calmer and safer now. We accept each other and are more familiar with our own and each other's personality, habits and traits."

She continued confidently, "I don't experience disappointment now the way I did a couple of years ago. I write in my journal most days and attempt to process my feelings, because I still have a lot of healing to do. I spend a lot of time with my best friend, Nancy," smiled Cinderella. "We both have a desire to understand our past, how it affects us and what to do about it. We support each other by listening to one another and sharing our journeys with each other. We never get tired of talking."

"What a relief," put in Charming. "Cindy gives me summaries of her insights and the books she reads, but now there's someone else to get the blow-by-blow descriptions. Believe it or not, though, I've read a few of the books myself."

"Good! I'm pleased," said Fairy Godmother. "I remember when you two were so unaware that you hurt each other without even realizing it. Guilt, shame, and blame were tools you used to control each other. And Cindy wanted the infatuation stage of your relationship to last forever."

"Yes, and what a revelation it was to realize that I didn't have to change Charming — that I could love him for who he truly is," commented Cinderella.

Charming nodded in agreement. "You don't know what a relief that is."

"You are both doing a very good job of living and relating from a base of unconditional love," said Fairy Godmother. "You are learning to recognize when either of you is being controlling and judgmental."

"I think your appraisal is too generous," remarked Charming. "Much of the time we do a good job, but it isn't easy. We have to work at it constantly. When I'm in a negative frame of mind, I still think it's much too hard and not worth the effort. When I retreat, several days may pass before we finally spend quality time together, allowing me to work through my feelings. I'm always grateful to have someone with whom to connect — someone who doesn't give up."

Cinderella smiled and added, "When we get too busy to talk, whether because of work or the children, we have to be jolted into recognizing our unhealthy behaviors and returning to the communication guidelines you provided. I'm looking forward to having it come automatically."

"Don't be concerned that it doesn't come easily," said Fairy Godmother. "It took you years to learn the old patterns and habits. They were modeled to you when you were children, so the behaviors are deeply ingrained. Give yourselves time to make the necessary changes. It may be years before the communication skills become automatic, but that doesn't matter. The important thing is that you both are willing to change."

"Listening to you, I don't feel so bad that we don't always practice everything we know," smiled Charming. "Sometimes just my tone of voice or choice of words hurts Cinderella's feelings, and I want to kick myself. Then I remember that I'm still in the process of learning and changing, so it's okay."

"Wonderful! Keep talking kindly to yourself," said Fairy Godmother with a wink.

"Our parenting methods have changed, too," added Cinderella. "Charming and I were parented very differently, so we frequently trigger each other with seemingly incompatible approaches. But we almost always talk things through after a disagreement and are working toward a more unified parenting style."

"Knowing more about myself has affected all of my relationships, even those at work," said Charming.

"What has been the greatest change in your relationship over the past two years?" asked Fairy Godmother.

Like eager pupils, Cinderella and Charming began to speak at once. Then Cinderella stopped and gave Charming the floor. She silently recalled how she used to complain about Charming's unwillingness to share. Now that he was willing, she wanted to give him the space to talk.

"The number one change is Nancy," said Charming. "Now that Cindy shares so much with her friend, I don't have to be her main support, which is good because it's not my strong suit. And the fact that Cindy is busy with work outside the castle takes additional pressure off of me," explained Charming.

"I have to admit that I don't miss him like I used to," laughed Cinderella.

"What change would you say has most influenced the relationship in the past two years?" asked Fairy Godmother.

Cinderella answered this time. "I would have to say getting in touch with and starting my life's spiritual work. Moving beyond traditional roles required taking many personal risks, and I don't think I could have done it without your support, Fairy Godmother. I'm no longer afraid to develop and share my talents."

Cinderella had solved the mystery of how to help her relationship. Her life no longer revolved around Charming. She had developed meaningful interests of her own. At the same time she enjoyed the richness of her life with Charming.

Cinderella and Charming elaborated further on the changes of the past two years. Afterwards, the three agreed to continue meeting occasionally, even when things were going well, just to ensure continued progress and peace. As Fairy Godmother was about to leave, Charming called her back.

"Oh, I almost forgot to tell you," exclaimed Charming. "I've started meeting with my Fairy Godfather. To hear him talk, he's got more lessons for me than a wizard has brews."

Fairy Godmother laughed. "I'll make a note to check his credentials," she teased.

Points to Ponder from Chapter Eleven

1. Committing to a relationship that is creative and continually evolving is vastly easier than committing to one that is static and boring.

   Once the issues of control and disappointment are faced, it is much easier to accept a partner's traits. Disappointment generated by your partner's failure to change or make you happy is replaced by appreciation for the relationship as a rich, creative milieu for the growth and development of both partners.

2. A good relationship nourishes the skills needed to build and maintain emotional closeness and the mutual support system for weathering the ups and downs of life.

   A good relationship is never perfect because individuals are never perfect. It evolves as the partners evolve and requires continuous attention.

3. It takes a long time to completely let go of controlling behavior and the tendency to be judgmental.

4. Some needs can be better met outside the relationship.

   For example, if one partner has a greater need to explore personal growth and awareness, it can be helpful to do so with a friend.

5. It is normal to feel at times that the relationship is not working or is too much trouble. Such feelings need to be honored.

   Use these experiences as catalysts for journal writing, therapy, attendance at a workshop or finding practical tips in a self-help book.

6. The more you know yourself, the more you improve all your relationships.

   You are responsible for your own growth and awareness. You are the leading character of your life script as well as the editor, director and scriptwriter.

Epilogue

Cinderella learned many things that changed her life while working with her spiritual teacher, Fairy Godmother. She learned that true happiness cannot come from another person. Being totally and unconditionally loved by another, pleasurable as it is, cannot be relied upon as a primary source of fulfillment.

Happiness, when experienced, is usually the result of a condition or event; it rarely causes the condition or event. True happiness must come from personal fulfillment. Cinderella's relationship with Charming improved as her consciousness evolved and she was able to heal the past, love herself, understand and clarify her perceptions, learn specific communication techniques, and begin to actualize her spiritual purpose.

As she felt more complete and balanced, Cinderella was less apt to look for happiness outside of herself, principally from Prince Charming. She began the creative process of actualizing her potential, concentrating first on inner work, and later on manifesting her potential in the outer world. She felt an emerging need to share talents beyond those of caregiver, the latter "talent" having developed from early conditioning in the service of her stepmother and stepsisters.

Living happily ever after is not dependent on outside circumstances, but on a shift in consciousness — hence, multiple endings are possible. Granted, many people prefer the ending in which the couple stay together and continue to work on the relationship and themselves. However, predetermining the "right" outcome of a spiritual journey is impossible, because the outcome develops from the awareness and consciousness of both partners.

With guidance beyond her own restricted frame of reference, Cinderella learned to expand her world. At the close of the story, she possessed a clearer understanding of the purpose of relationships. Cinderella learned that relationships provoke the emergence of unresolved patterns from the past, which must then be transformed. Once she understood this process, Cinderella was able to recognize when she was projecting her own issues onto Prince Charming and when he was projecting his onto her.

In the second ending, both partners developed the ability to recognize and alleviate projections, and to take responsibility for their own actions, perceptions and responses. They learned new communication skills that enabled them to more safely risk mutual confrontation and thus resolve conflict. They went on to build a solid relationship with mature love based on trust, respect, equality and emotional intimacy.

Continuous self-improvement is an important component of any loving, growing, creative relationship, and requires the dedication of both partners. While Cinderella chose to devote a significant amount of time to the inner healing and expansion of her awareness, she allowed Charming to proceed at his own pace. She found fulfillment in developing her talents and she wanted to make the world a better place. Her self-esteem grew as she continued to heal, take risks, love herself and connect to the Source of her being. Cinderella learned to live beyond the restrictive belief that happiness depended on Prince Charming. By moving beyond the Prince Charming fantasy, Cinderella learned to live happily ever after.

Notes

Notes